DR. BOB'S PATIENTS SHARE THEIR RESULTS

Most impactful of what I have learned from Dr. Bob is the importance of eating the foods that help my body to heal. Since following Dr. Bob's advice, the pain I have experienced for so long is gone and I continue to get stronger every day with more energy. I also was an MS patient, but since receiving regular care from Dr. Bob, I have had less active lesions every year and my last MRI showed zero activity.

The pain in my body has been dramatically reduced. I've still had the occasional birthday cake, and when I have sugar now I feel the difference! During the past two years, I have lost a total of 20 pounds without even really trying; I've just made healthier food choices. I recently had a yearly physical and all of my blood work came back at good levels. My cholesterol levels have improved to a normal range.

I feel that meeting Dr. Bob was truly a blessing. I am grateful for all he has done to help improve my health!

—Brady R.

I used to take at least 1,500 Tylenol a year and get frequent ear and sinus infections. By getting regular adjustments from Dr. Bob and eating right, I haven't had Tylenol in over 12 years. The pain in my body has been reduced 100 percent and my energy has increased. After 30 years of marriage, our intimate life is still going strong. If you just try Dr. Bob's suggestions, I think you will be amazed by what he knows and how much he really does care about you.

—David W.

D0711710

I had lost weight and gained it back every year for nearly 14 years. Recently, I made a lifestyle change and finally implemented what Dr. Bob had instructed me to do over that time frame. Within five months, I shed 65 pounds. Dr. Bob had mentioned to me that for every pound I was overweight I added 200 miles of blood vessels. I can truly say that my heart doesn't have to pump that additional 13,000 miles anymore.

Also, my blood pressure got out of control. With my lifestyle changes and weight reduction, I was able to get the blood pressure back in line without the use of prescription drugs. My overall energy has gone from sluggish to high and I now experience more energy and stamina in my intimate life.

Dr. Bob actually saved my life. It took a while for me to totally get on board with what he was teaching and encouraging me to do for my personal health and diet. Now that I have made the lifestyle changes in my diet and exercise routine, I feel like I am 18 again. I literally feel 30 years younger. I know that by staying the course with Dr. Bob's recommendations, I am going to live a healthier, fuller life and be around for my wife and our children and someday their children.

—Doug B.

I have learned many things from Dr. Bob. I had previously been taking aspirin and garlic pills to reduce my cholesterol. Dr. Bob suggested a reduced-carb diet would help lower my cholesterol and it did—by 30 points! He also stressed how important the right diet is for good health, especially reducing sugar. Since following Dr. Bob's suggestions, I've been maintaining a strong immune system and a drug-free life. I would say that a healthier life is a better life! I appreciate having an excellent resource in Dr. Bob for maintaining a healthy lifestyle.

—Pat D.

Since becoming a regular patient of Dr. Bob, I have discovered that optimal health is realized when one combines three things: spinal corrective care, a healthful nutritional approach to diet and a nurturing of spiritual health. Through 24 years of Dr. Bob's care and professional advice, I have gone from a 40-year-old with chronic back trouble (with the medical community pushing for surgery) to a stable condition that allowed me to reach retirement age with increased energy. My lumbar back pain is old history and my neck pain has been eliminated. I also lost about 15 pounds and have kept it off. My red blood cell count has gone up, which lowered my risk of anemia.

My previous medical doctors had me on 2 mg of Ativan® per day for 15 years. After learning how bad that was for my liver, I've been able to wean off of it and am down to .50 mg per day. My admiration for Dr. Bob and his family of caregivers is very high. I especially like that he practices what he preaches!

—Larry D.

After receiving consistent spinal adjustments from Dr. Bob, my energy level has dramatically increased. He has also taught me how sugar affects my body much more than I realized. Now I am far more aware of what I eat, no longer eating desserts or sweets. As a result, my sinuses are a lot better, my back pain is completely gone (yes, there is a correlation) and I've lost 18 pounds without even trying. My intimate life has gone from an 8 out of 10 to 11! I feel great!

—Paul G.

Dr. Bob has taught me the importance of Celtic Sea Salt® and iodine (which does not include table salt). Iodine can help assist the thyroid gland to function normally. Dr. Bob has also taught me how sugar creates such havoc on the body. My health has changed for the better by following Dr. Bob's recommendations. For example, I recently was exposed to a chemical that creates respiratory problems. Dr. Bob recommended some dietary supplementation that has been improving my respiratory situation. Dr. Bob has also helped assist me to create a better functioning thyroid through dietary supplementation. The hardest recommendation to follow is "no eating sugar." I still have not achieved this goal 100 percent of the time; however, I have dramatically reduced my sugar consumption. Furthermore, I have noticed that my immune system is stronger when I do not consume sugar. Let's not forget that Dr. Bob is also a chiropractor. Therefore, my chance of developing arthritis is minimized by getting adjustments regularly. When I tie this all together, Dr. Bob has been helping me do what I asked him to do—to achieve optimal health.

If you follow everything Dr. Bob says, there is no reason to have pain. I am pain free with increased energy levels. If you follow Dr. Bob's recommendations, your mind clarity will also improve.

—Jeff R.

Dr. Bob has taught me the importance of a balanced diet. As a result, my bodily pain has reduced tremendously, I have felt consistently healthy and my body moves smoothly without any stiff joints, and I have lost weight. I have also noticed an increased amount of energy—I am not fatigued anymore. I just love the fact that I can be healthy without medications! I'm amazed at how Dr. Bob has tied it all together, proving to me that our bodies have the inherent ability to heal themselves. I do know, however, that I need to keep up my optimal living habits if I want stay at this level.

—Andrew S.

Dr. Bob is constantly teaching his patients about proper postural alignment and the importance of diet. After following Dr. Bob's suggestions, I have more energy and the pain in my lower back has been greatly reduced. I have lost weight and increased muscle tone. My mate and I have more energy for all activities. Dr. Bob has helped me tremendously!

—Craig M.

The fact that you're reading this book indicates a genuine desire on your part to acquire the necessary information that, when applied, will result in a marked improvement in your health and overall quality of life. As a critical thinker, you may have a reasonable suspicion of our food and of our blatantly misnamed "health care industry." Our "disease management" industry would be more accurate. Let's face it: If we're not sick, they're out of business. So congratulations—you're on the right track to a better life!

I've been a patient of Dr. Bob's for years, and with regular spinal adjustments have experienced relief from neck and shoulder pain and numbness in my thumb and forefinger along with increased strength and mobility. His continued commitment to education has helped me make dietary adjustments resulting in weight loss, increased energy and improved circulation and a bolstered immune system. I rarely, if ever, get sick.

I'm grateful for the improvements in my life that are a direct result of the application of the knowledge I've received. However, there are times when I've endured the negative effects resulting from my failure to apply what I've learned from Dr. Bob. I much prefer the former. Procrastination fertilizes fear. Action eliminates it! Dr. Bob gives you the knowledge you need to take the action that will dramatically improve your health.

—Kevin G.

Dr. Bob's

MEN'S HEALTH — THE BASICS

Dr. Robert DeMaria
The Drugless Doctor

Drugless Doctor™ LLC
Elyria, OH

Dr.Bob's MEN'S HEALTH — THE BASICS

by Robert DeMaria, D.C., N.H.D.

Published by:
Drugless Doctor™ LLC
362 East Bridge Street
Elyria, OH 44035

Phone: **(440) 323-3841**
Fax:: **(440) 323-1566**
E-Mail: **DrBob@Druglessdoctor.com**
Website: **www.druglessdoctor.com**

ISBN: 978-0-9728907-6-2

Printed in the United States of America

0 9 8 7 6 5 4 3 2 1

DISCLAIMER

This information is provided with the understanding that the author is not liable for the misconception or misuse of information included. Every effort has been made to make this material as complete and accurate as possible. The author of this material shall have neither liability nor responsibility to any person or entity with respect to any loss, damage or injury caused or alleged to be caused directly or indirectly by the information contained in this manuscript. The information presented herein is not intended to be a substitute for medical counseling.

Book Cover design by Ariel Vergez of Vujà Dé Studios, LLC

Page design by Peri Poloni-Gabriel, Knockout Design, www.knockoutbooks.com

CONTENTS

ACKNOWLEDGMENTS

We are living in an age where technology has absorbed what appears to be every precious extra moment of our day, using up all the time we might otherwise spend engaging in exercise and other optimal health pursuits. So many men come into my clinical practice having lived a life of reckless abandon but are now hoping to return to normal with an easy potion or two, believing that they have somehow been granted the same nine lives and extended warranties found in the video games they enjoy playing. I want to recognize and give kudos to all the men who have lived this way in the past but have now made the wise and unselfish decision to not only change and improve their own health but also impact the health of their families and loved ones. I am seeing more and more men with a newfound health consciousness who want to get better and even read books; without you, I would not have a purpose for putting this information to paper.

Every day there are people who cross my path and impact my life in some way or another. I'd like to thank them here. I want to especially acknowledge the team I have been so fortunate to organize for taking this material to the world, helping men to live a healthier life without the dependence and side effects of medication. My sons, Dominic and Anthony, have always been a huge support and part of my motivation to conquer the world by being "The Drugless Doctor." My hat goes off to Dominic and his team for motivating me to speed into the social media age with a new brand and new information. Thank you, Vujà Dé Studios.

I must say the most significant person impacting every move of my life is my wife, Debbie. We have been "an item" since we were kids in high school. Without her support and keen insight, I would not be here to give you this timely information.

My prayer is for each and every one of you to create and live the life of your dreams. Thank you in advance for passing what you have learned here on to your inner circle of friends and family.

FOREWORD

BY DOMINIC DEMARIA

To most people, my dad is simply known as Dr. Bob. Growing up, my brother, Anthony, and I were often asked what it was like to have Dr. Bob as a father, with our response usually leaning toward, "It's okay." After all, whose father doesn't get up at 4:30 a.m. every day, pray with their spouse, make breakfast and lunch (for himself and my mom), guest-spot on a few morning radio shows, host a TV program, run two businesses, prepare for a seminar, work on a book to help millions of people, go to sleep and wake up and do it all over again the next day? Well, apparently not many fathers, something Anthony and I later found out.

As I have matured (I'm now approaching the big 3-0), the "It's okay" has turned into elevated gratitude and unrivaled respect. After I graduated with my bachelor's degree, I worked at my father's practice and witnessed firsthand patients who would come in with all their various shapes, sizes, ailments, odors and walking devices. The crazy part was, they would get better. Not by my dad writing a prescription, but by him getting to know them, personalizing a road map to their individual health, suggesting lifestyle changes and adjusting their subluxations.

After I graduated with my MBA I needed to write a thesis, and after *really* not wanting to return to Ohio, I was presented with the opportunity to write the 100-page colossus on my father as a brand. (For everyone into self-branding, by the way, this was before the whole "yourself as a brand" craze.) Throughout those three months, I noticed that the world, not just the United States, was in need of a health hero. Not someone who suggested taking a pill to make it feel better while adding countless side effects. Does anyone really want painful or frequent urination? Rather someone who believed in health the way that health and life should be; hence, "The Drugless Doctor" came into existence.

Today, I find myself heeding the call to encourage everyone to listen, read and apply my dad's content. This book, centering on men's health, is so relevant for men today—no matter what demographic you find yourself. I'm glad that Dr. Bob has decided to address and provide practical solutions to modern-day concerns that are being neglected in many health conversations across the country and globe. Having built up "Dr. Bob: The Drugless Doctor" as the archetypal health hero, I want to encourage you (because you are reading this book for a reason) that you *can* be healthy, but it will require change and responsibility on your part. Not to worry; you're in good shape because there's someone here to help guide you along the way. #goodthings

@DominicDeMaria
@VujaDeStudios

INTRODUCTION

As a practicing drugless doctor since 1978, I am very concerned about the toxic health crisis occurring in America that is impacting our basic essentials: water, food, air and soil. I always try to focus on the positive, but what's actually going on needs to be addressed. Our children are exposed to chemicals from before birth, the negative health consequences from stress are explosive, broken marriages with family discord are common, financial upheaval has sabotaged the once stable environment in our country with an impact on all layers, creating a new level of working poor. Nearly every facet of the world has been affected in some way by terrorism. We have a health care crisis looming without a trustworthy ambassador focusing on achieving optimal well-being. All of these concerns have started to take their toll on the foundational health of men, the physical pillar of our society.

I never once in my career surmised that I would write a book focusing primarily on men, discussing health issues that focus on the basics: low testosterone, hormonal health, pain syndromes, cholesterol, fat metabolism, weight loss and erectile dysfunction. I sometimes have a challenge wrapping my brain around the fact that some men require a prescription medication to arrive at an erection when this is so basic to our human existence. How far have we deteriorated as a culture to require so many medications just to survive day to day—drugs for sleep, pain and depression, high cholesterol, high blood pressure, digestive distress, sinus infections and toe nail fungus? How can we as a society, a group of educated people, allow ourselves to be one of the unhealthiest nations on the planet while spending the most money on health care? There is a serious problem here that needs addressing, and I, for one, plan on doing it.

"Drugless therapeutics" is an integral part of my clinical chiropractic practice and my life. I have been trained and tested in drugless therapeutics, including a Fellow in Spinal Engineering and a Diplomat Certification in Orthopedics, and have a Doctor of Natural Health diploma. The information you have in your hand is a compilation of time-tested protocols, recommendations and experience from over three decades of clinical experience—from having worked literally in the trenches since the 1970s—examining, treating and consulting with many thousands of new patients in hundreds of thousands of office visits. I engage daily in important dialogue to assist my anxious new patients to get to the cause of their symptoms and then create a strategy to restore optimal health.

This book, then, focuses on common conditions men deal with every day. Men historically, from my experience, do not like to go to doctors, and today's educated male researches his symptoms and body signals on the Internet, in health magazines and traditional medical research institutions' portals since he doesn't necessarily feel confident with the conventional Western physician. Men today do not want to go into a room with someone who is in a hurry to write a prescription and/or suggest a list of tests. I know this is true because I confront my male patients with this question: "Do you have a doctor you feel confident with?" Most of the time they look at me and admit that they are in my office because of an issue that is not getting better and they want to address it by getting to the root cause, something their conventional doctor is not offering to do. Many want a drugless solution.

Therefore, I am excited for you to have found this information—it will positively impact you, whatever your age and current state of health. I have been around the race track of life many times and, just like you, have the scars to show it. I am a post-WWII baby boomer with two grown sons and aging parents who have since passed. I am self-employed and have been married for more than 35 years. I'm not looking for anyone's approval, so I really don't mince words; I call it and say it like it is.

I have specifically written this book for you, the guy on the couch or on the golf course who wants to change but just doesn't yet know what to do. Let me make it really easy. This book is about getting healthy from the inside out. I have divided the book into a sequence of chapters that focus on the most common health challenges I see and respond to with drugless care. I am going to give you simple "Action Steps" at the end of each chapter for improving your health in that area. Yes, you will need to make some changes, but let's go slow. Don't throw anything out; don't get frustrated. You will have everything you need to get healthy from your own grocery store.

Let's do health together!

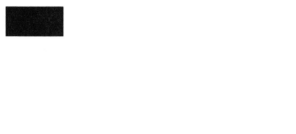

1

HORMONES 101

Every part of your body is integrally connected to every other part. The key to this connection, and to your daily function, is the hormonal or endocrine system. As men, we don't normally think about our hormones very much. We tend to be far more aware of what is going on with the hormones of our female friends or mate. So it may come as a surprise that we will be discussing your hormone levels at length in this book. Yes, men have varying hormone levels and they are impacted by food choices, toxins and stress, just like in their female counterparts. In fact, in my practice I am noticing more each passing week that the male hormones in men are falling to levels that create fatigue, pain, low libido and depression. I know that the nuggets you will learn glean in this chapter and in this book will assist you in making wise choices and developing strategies for optimal health—improving the quality of your life without taking any more medications. Trust me when I tell you that life can once again be grand. So, let's get started!

Hormones act as messengers in the body, and the endocrine (or glandular) system plays a critical role in muscle strength, blood sugar levels, sexual desire and the ability to respond physically to those needs. The endocrine system is made up of eight different glands located strategically throughout the body.

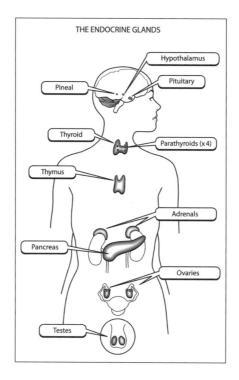

In addition to these major glands, the endocrine system includes pockets of hormone-producing cells in the small intestines, heart, kidneys and stomach. The endocrine glands and other systems work together to maintain health and, in particular, proper sexual function.

HYPOTHALAMUS

The hypothalamus is the CEO of the hormonal system and the commander-in-chief of all hormonal activity. It responds to all sorts of stimuli, from your five senses and even your thoughts and emotions, and it is in control of all of your body functions—directing glands and tissues in what to do (for example, directing saliva glands to secrete when you think of food, chill bumps on the arms when there is a cool breeze, increasing your heart rate when you start to run, and so on). When your body is under any type of stress, the hypothalamus responds by sending instructions to other parts of the brain and body on what to do. The hypothalamus connects the emotional mind to the physical man. When you think about a past or future event and get a "pit" in your stomach, it is because your hypothalamus is processing the event. This is one of the ways stress impacts your physiology. And, interestingly, while it may feel as though sexual needs originate in your body, sex actually starts in the mind. Most men are initially stimulated visually, while women become aware of sexual feelings as a response to romantic thoughts and gestures. These sights and feelings arouse the emotions, and the hypothalamus releases hormones to activate other glands in the body, connecting sexual thoughts with physical responses to ready the body for sexual intimacy.

TESTES

Testes are a pair of reproductive glands found in males. They are cradled in the scrotum and hang outside of the body, where they produce sperm and testosterone. The term "gonad" refers to testes in males.

ADRENAL

You have two adrenal glands, one located on the top of each kidney. They serve many functions, including affecting the size of the pupils of the eyes, being instrumental in the ability to ejaculate in men, and producing steroids including sex hormones, pain-relieving cortisol and mineral-regulating ligament-strengthening hormones. I often see patients whose adrenal glands are overworked and exhausted. A common body signal of this exhaustion is sensitivity to bright light. Wearing sunglasses because of adrenal stress prevents the full spectrum of light from reaching the back of the eye, complicating your optimal health puzzle.

PANCREAS

The pancreas produces insulin and enzymes for proper digestion and metabolism and can be overworked when the diet is full of processed foods. Packaged, devitalized foods have been stripped of nutrients, resulting in increased stress on the pancreas to make up for insufficient enzyme levels.

THYROID AND PARATHYROID

The thyroid receives messages from the pituitary gland and creates thyroid hormones, which are used by all the cells of the body. The thyroid sets the pace for optimal metabolism. The parathyroid works in conjunction with the thyroid to aid in proper calcium metabolism.

PINEAL

This tiny gland is incredibly significant but rarely discussed by health care professionals. It is linked to the hypothalamus and is influenced by diet and nutrition. The pineal gland produces and secretes melatonin in response to light rays from the sun and those reflected off the moon, creating the cycle of waking and sleeping.

I've consulted many patients who struggle with a condition called seasonal affective disorder, or SAD, which closely mimics depression. This disorder occurs late in summer, as the seasons change and the hours of daylight rapidly decline. These patients also experience emotional struggles at this time of year as their children are starting kindergarten, older children are returning to school or teens are heading off to college or are otherwise leaving the nest. The combination of emotional challenges and changing sleep and wake cycles can be overwhelming, and I've found SAD to be a result of these struggles as well as stress and nutritional deficiencies. It's very common for these patients to experience a decreased sex drive as well. If you are suffering this way, I recommend using a product called phosphatidylcholine and taking up to nine per day. Phosphatidylcholine is very useful in stabilizing emotional health when challenged in the fall by seasonal affective disorder.

PITUITARY

The pituitary gland is nearly as significant as the hypothalamus. Once it receives orders from the CEO, it conveys the messages to several glands and tissues critical to all hormonal functions, including the testes, adrenal glands and thyroid. The pituitary also plays a major role in metabolism, digestion and growth by influencing the autonomic nervous system.

My hope is that, after taking a closer look at these glands, you will realize how amazing and important your endocrine system is. Thoughts would never become manifest were it not for this system of hormone messengers preparing your body for action. Unfortunately, I see an epidemic of patients whose endocrine systems are overworked, stressed and nutritionally starving. When a patient complains of a lack of energy and displays overall poor health and a reduction in sexual desire, it's almost always because their endocrine system is exhausted and near collapse. Other symptoms of hormonal burnout include chronic degenerative diseases like diabetes, high blood pressure and whole-body inflammation with elevated cholesterol. These three conditions alone are responsible for most of the asexual marriages and resulting marital challenges I've treated.

I use various assessment forms in my practice to help my patients restore optimal health, and what I have observed is a pattern of exhaustion and hormonal dysfunction in men with back pain, headache and shoulder and other joint pains. These same individuals, whom I see plenty of in my practice, quietly admit to decreased or non-existent sexual desire and erectile dysfunction complications. It's been my experience that most of these men are physically exhausted—drained from poor diets, over-indulging in alcohol, abusing recreational and prescription drugs, smoking cigarettes and experiencing daily pressure from their jobs. Many of them are taking one or more psychoactive prescription medications just to take the edge off.

THE IMPORTANCE OF DIET

Your body makes hormones from the food you eat. Healthful, organic, whole foods result in healthy hormone production. Conversely, toxic foods full of sugar, taste enhancers, preservatives and trans fats will result in inadequate hormone production and a body that is literally starving for nutrition. You, too, may be suffering from hormonal imbalance and lowered libido, and the reason is likely as close as your kitchen pantry. If you are consuming a diet full of nutritionally deficient processed foods and are addicted to sweets, soft drinks and calorie-laden meals, your body is doing its best with what you're feeding it, but it's not functioning anywhere close to its peak!

The endocrine system is probably the first part of your body to be impacted by nutritional deficiencies. I often notice that sexual functions, which are so important to men, are affected just as much by nutrition as they are by physical and emotional health. Thankfully, nutritional changes are relatively simple to make and the effects are almost immediate. Instead of masking sexual problems by taking prescription drugs (and causing a whole host of side effects that then must be dealt with), you can radically improve your health and the sexual health of your relationship or marriage by making small changes in your diet and lifestyle.

If you recognize some of the symptoms of hormonal exhaustion discussed in this chapter, I strongly suggest you read Chapter 13 on the adrenal system and commit to making healthy changes in your diet and lifestyle. Your body will thank you, your sex drive will increase and you and your spouse or significant other will find renewed passion and excitement as you travel this journey toward health and healing together.

HORMONES 101 – ACTION STEPS

- ☐ Your endocrine system requires whole foods to operate at top efficiency. Start eliminating processed foods from your diet and get your nutrients from organic, whole foods.

- ☐ Organic high lignan flax oil is a great way to start improving overall hormonal health. You should take one tablespoon per 100 pounds of your body weight.

- ☐ Eliminate sugar from your diet to avoid stressing the adrenal glands.

- ☐ Plan your meals with the entire family and eat together as often as possible to create healthy eating habits in your children that will last a lifetime.

2

BALANCING MALE HORMONES

The balance of male hormones is not as intricate as what is going on in a female's body. The primary concern for males is the cholesterol-originating chart I have included in Chapter 13 on adrenal health. Testosterone can be sourced from cholesterol like the other steroid hormones can. As touched upon in Chapter 1 in our discussions of the adrenal glands and diet, when men have stress in their daily lives, they will have impaired adrenal function. In this state, all the nutrients for cellular function will be used to make cortisone to handle the stress and very little will be left over to make testosterone. In this deficiency mode, men lose their desire for sexual intimacy; in other words, they can have decreased libido. This is a common complaint that I see on the symptom survey form I use in my office when initiating the whole-body assessment of male patients. A lack of sexual desire coincides with a run-down endocrine, or hormone, system. It is as if the spark plugs do not have any fuel to spark. The way the body operates, the nutrients needed to encourage sexual arousal are being used for you to survive.

The following scenario is one I see in my office on a regular basis. My most challenging patient to treat and educate is the male between

25 and 45 years old. They think they still have the testosterone and ability of a 19-year-old, but in actuality most have the body of a 55-year-old! They are at the point in life where work can be very stressful and where many financial responsibilities (such as college tuition, larger houses and "toy" payments like boat, vacation house and club fees) are coming into reality.

The weekly recorded diet journals of my male patients reveal anything but good nutritional habits. Food on the run, along with a night or weekend out with the guys, promotes nothing healthy but the size of their waistline. Cholesterol runs high with this type of lifestyle; the serum cholesterol readings are near the price of gasoline. The result is that you just do not feel well.

The pressures of downsizing at work and the fear of a future that is unknown create the physiology that generates far too many demands on the entire body, including your immune and hormonal function. Before you know it, your doctor is handing you prescriptions for blood pressure and cholesterol medications, a "mild" antidepressant and a new pill to promote an erection. Sound too far out? Not really. I hear about this type of consultation from my male patients consistently. One of the best things you can do is to eat the foods suggested in Chapter 17 on the Page Fundamental Diet Plan. If not, you will suffer with a loss of sexual desire and overall poor health.

UNDERSTANDING MALE HORMONES

To really take command of your health, it's an advantage to have some sense of what is going on in the physiology of your hormones. I promise to keep this as simple as possible.

Male hormones are called androgens. "Androgen" is the generic term for any natural or synthetic compound, usually a steroid hormone, which stimulates or controls the development and maintenance of masculine characteristics in vertebrates by binding to androgen receptors. This includes the activity of the accessory male sex organs and development of male secondary sex characteristics. Androgens, which were first discovered in 1936, are also called androgenic hormones or testoids. Androgens are also the original anabolic steroids. They are also the precursor of all estrogens, the female sex hormones. The primary and most well-known androgen is testosterone.

Testosterone is a steroid hormone from the androgen group. Testosterone is primarily secreted in the testes of males and the ovaries of females, although small amounts are secreted by the adrenal glands. It is the principal male sex hormone and an anabolic steroid. In both males and females, it plays key roles in health and well-being, such as in enhancing libido, energy and immune function as well as protecting against osteoporosis. Males produce more testosterone than females do. On average, the adult male body produces about 20 to 30 times the amount produced by an adult female's body.

Conversely, the human hormone estrogen is produced in greater amounts by females, less so by males. Testosterone causes the appearance of masculine traits (e.g., deepening voice, pubic and facial hairs, muscular build, etc.). Women, like men, rely on testosterone to maintain libido, bone density and muscle mass throughout their lives.

A subset of androgens is the adrenal androgens, which include any of the steroids synthesized by the adrenal cortex, the outer portion of the adrenal gland. These function as weak steroids, or steroid precursors, and include dehydroepiandrosterone (DHEA). DHEA is a steroid hormone produced from cholesterol in the adrenal cortex and is the primary precursor of the natural estrogen, androstenedione (known as "Andro"), an androgenic steroid produced by the testes, adrenal cortex and ovaries. While androstenediones are converted metabolically to testosterone and other androgens, they are also the parent structure of estrone, one of three naturally occurring estrogens. Use of androstenedione as an athletic or body-building supplement has been banned by the International Olympic Committee as well as other sporting organizations.

Because of the tremendous effect of stress on the hormonal system, I advise all of my male patients to limit their responsibilities and obligations where possible. Of course, this is easier said than done! Optimal health is all about prioritizing. When I was helping to raise our sons, I stopped or limited most of my extracurricular activities, such as community organization and church commitments, sports events and time with "the guys," as I did not want to burn out my adrenal glands. Also, as a family, we lived within our budget. A saying I find value in remembering is, "Your earning power never satisfies your yearning desire." Try to minimize your desire for consumption. You won't have to work so hard, which will mean less stress. And less stress over finances equals less stress at home, as financial concerns are one of the leading causes of American divorces.

A FEW SECRET WEAPONS

Now I'd like to share with you a few secret weapons for protecting your hormone health. The first is iodine supplementation. Men need iodine, as do women. Men who have prostate swelling and/ or elevated PSA (prostate screening) readings will be pleasantly surprised when those levels go down over time with iodine use. I encourage a regular supply of Celtic Sea Salt®, as it is a great source of iodine. Have your doctor give you a requisition for an assessment to determine your iodine function and a T3, T4 and TSH panel for thyroid function. A urine iodine test is also helpful. Recommendations will be based on your lab results. For many of my male patients, I have advised taking up to 12 mg a day of organic iodine, in tablet or capsule form. In fact, that's how much I personally supplement each day.

A second secret weapon for men and women alike is to check your torso, legs and arms for small, raised, red-cherry, bead-like bumps, officially called "cherry hemangiomas." An abundance of these little bumps is a sign that there may be estrogen saturation. When men have too much estrogen, they can have prostate issues. A leading factor that increases estrogen in the body is eating conventional meat, rather than organic. While I understand that budgets can be limited, the benefit to prostate health makes organic meats worth saving for. Soy is the other culprit. Soy increases estrogen in men. For this reason alone, I do not promote soy products. Men do not ever need to put an estrogen type of product in their body; it can create a swollen prostate gland.

I am now discovering a near epidemic of men over 55 who actually have more estrogen in their system than women do. I know this reversal may seem a bit farfetched, but it is occurring! There is a little-known fact that testosterone can be flipped over to estrogen because of an enzyme called aromatase. If you are noticing that your breasts are enlarging and that you are becoming a bit more passive, you may want to investigate an aromatase inhibitor. I use a natural product in my practice for men who have prostate challenges and decreased libido.

My third recommendation is zinc. Both men and women can be negatively impacted by a deficiency of this essential mineral. I generally see a diminished sense of taste and smell in those who do not have a sufficient amount. Memory loss, slow healing, white spots on the nails and impaired insulin function can also be precipitated by a zinc deficiency. Additionally, men need zinc for the prostate to function—this is critical. Eating wheat and soy products will deplete zinc, as does sugar and stress. I highly recommend getting a bottle of the Zinc Taste Test, which you can get at most health food stores or through a natural health care provider, to identify any potential zinc situation you may have.

Now, before moving on to my final tips, I'd like you to review what you've read so far.

BALANCING MALE HORMONES – ACTION STEPS

☐ For optimal testosterone levels, aim for less stress and eliminate sugar from your diet.

☐ Focus on eating protein and non-starchy veggies versus sweet fruits—bananas, raisins and grapes—which stress the adrenal gland.

☐ Have a tissue-hair mineral analysis, which may show a zinc deficiency and should be treated accordingly. Avoid wheat and soy if your zinc levels are low.

☐ For optimal hormone health, take one tablespoon of a quality source of omega-3 flax oil a day per 100 pounds of body weight.

☐ An important protocol for male patients includes support for the pituitary, adrenal and orchic (testes) glands. As such, it is wise to take some type of liver support (we'll discuss this in Chapter 8), flax oil and iodine. I also recommend taking a full-spectrum oil, such as black currant seed capsules, and folic acid B12, which helps the creation of adequately sized red blood cells. I follow a protocol like this, which helps keep my endocrine system at an optimal level.

☐ I used to have a lot of cherry hemangiomas, which went away many years ago when I stopped consuming alcohol. Greatly limit your intake or cut it out altogether.

☐ Men should not ever use soy products.

☐ If you notice that your breasts are enlarging, I would encourage a Saliva Hormone Assessment to check your testosterone levels. Go to **www.druglessdoctor.com** under the Client Services/ Testing Services link for details. If you notice your estrogen is elevated, consider an aromatase inhibitor.

NOTES

3

ATTACK HEART ATTACKS AND HIGH BLOOD PRESSURE

You need only read the obituary page in your local newspaper to see that there are more people passing on today in their 30s and 40s from a "short illness" (i.e., heart attack) than at any other time in history. Heart disease is, in fact, one of the leading causes of death in the Western world. So, what is going on?

SOME IMPORTANT QUESTIONS

To begin to answer that, let me first ask you a few questions that will reveal to you your own understanding of heart health. Then I'd like to answer these common concerns one by one, from a Drugless Doctor's perspective and experience.

- What causes a heart attack?
- Can people of normal weight have a heart attack?
- Can people taking cholesterol-lowering medications get a heart attack?

- Are beef and cheese the primary reasons blood vessels get plugged?
- Is margarine a healthy alternative to butter?

Not sure? Let's take a look.

What Causes a Heart Attack?

The exact cause of heart attacks is not necessarily known. While there is much speculation, the answer you get will largely depend on what drug or medical supply company paid for the "research" into the issue, as the results are often skewed to create a platform for recommending the medication or services they are promoting. In the game of heart medicine, the competition is fierce and the monetary stakes high. Yet, the bottom line with the more popular medications and procedures, including angioplasties and stents, is that their positive impact on long-term heart health is very, very small—in fact, only 3 percent! Treatments based on the theory that vessels plugged from the accumulation of cholesterol causes heart attacks are not stopping heart attacks and heart disease from being one of the primary causes of death. People with years of normal cholesterol levels have heart attacks, so obviously something else must be going on here.

Can People of Normal Weight Have a Heart Attack?

There is no doubt that obesity's negative effect on health is stagger-ing. Many common causes of death, including cancer and diabetes, can be precipitated by having more tissue for the body to tend to. Yet, while being overweight certainly does nothing to promote life, the fact is that a person of any size can have a heart attack. I have observed people who are thin, fortunate to be blessed with what ap-pears to be a fast metabolism, become disabled due to heart health issues. These issues are caused by eating with reckless abandon those inflammation-inducing convenience and fast foods filled with "low-fat" ingredients with sugar and trans fat. Many heart patients also smoke, thereby bombarding all tissues of the body with thousands of poisonous toxins.

Can People Taking Cholesterol-Lowering Medications Get a Heart Attack?

It is now commonly accepted by those in the health field who are in the know that cholesterol is not the only culprit in heart attacks, as once believed. We now know that inflammation plays a major role in the restriction of blood flow to heart muscle. Heart muscle demands an uninterrupted flow of oxygen. Inflammation is precipitated by common foods that are loaded with sugar and trans fat. Over 150 pounds of sugar are consumed per person in the United States every year. Eight billion pounds of trans fat, or partially hydrogenated oils, are produced yearly in the U.S., 5 billion of which are used by the restaurant industry alone. The average American eats over 225 meals out of the home per year. Partially hydrogenated oils are also ravenously consumed in the form of snack and convenience items. These inflammation-generating foods are the leading factors causing heart challenges. So, yes, people taking cholesterol-lowering medications can get a heart attack.

Inflammation and heart health can be screened and assessed by having your C-reactive protein, or CRP, and homocysteine levels (we'll talk about this in a moment) evaluated. These two tests can assist your health care provider in determining your possibilities for potential heart challenges.

Are Beef and Cheese the Primary Reasons Blood Vessels Get "Plugged"?

After the Great Depression, a part of the American dream included having a chicken in every pot and roast beef and gravy every Sunday. Little thought was given to how the new American passion for food might at some point be a factor negatively impacting our health. An epidemic began to surface in the late 1950s with the acceleration of heart disease and heart attacks and has continued to this day, with heart disease being the leading cause of death. At first the culprit was thought to be cholesterol levels, but in spite of the public awareness to watch their dairy, red meat and cholesterol and a subsequent reduction in these obvious cholesterol-laden foods, the epidemic has continued to accelerate. So, what have we missed? What else might be causing the problem? As I have been alluding to, in this chapter I will show you that the leading factors creating heart disease are the very foods the scientific community told you to eat over the last 30 or 40 years—the low-fat diet with high levels of trans fat and sugar, synthetic oils and processed foods. These are the actual major causative factors of heart disease. The real good news here is that you can change your destiny for heart problems regardless of your family history by stopping the inflammation in your system.

Is Margarine a Healthy Alternative to Butter?

For years, margarine was promoted to be safer and better than butter because it did not have cholesterol in its makeup. Those "You can't fool Mother Nature" advertisements have had most Americans, to this day, deathly afraid of a mere tab of butter. But the truth is that margarine has NEVER been safe or good! Originally made with partially hydrogenated oil (trans fat), margarine is not even a food. Finally, in 1998, the negative facts about trans fat and partially hydrogenated oil came to public light, bringing some illumination on the subject. As it turns out, with its trans fat, margarine not only raises the LDL (bad) cholesterol, but it also lowers the HDL (good) cholesterol. The LDL cholesterol elevates with more inflammation, while the HDL cholesterol is depressed by trans fat—the opposite of what we need to have a healthy heart system. Were you duped? I'll bet yes! If so, you certainly weren't alone.

A QUICK LESSON IN HEART PHYSIOLOGY

The heart is a muscle that needs quality nutrients to function properly. The normal heart is a strong, muscular pump that moves blood continuously through the circulatory system. Each day the average heart beats 100,000 times and transports about 2,000 gallons of blood through the body. In a 70-year lifetime, an average human heart beats more than 2.5 *billion* times.

The circulatory system is the network of resilient tubes that carries blood throughout the body. It includes the heart, lungs, arteries, small arteries, and very tiny blood vessels. These blood vessels carry oxygen- and nutrient-rich blood to all parts of the body. The circulatory system also includes small veins and larger veins. These are the blood vessels that carry waste products and nutrient-depleted blood back to the heart and lungs. If all these vessels were laid end-to-end, they would extend about 60,000 miles—enough to encircle Earth more than two times!

The circulating blood transports oxygen and nutrients to all the body's organs and tissues, including the heart itself. It also picks up waste products from the body's cells. These waste products are removed as they're filtered through the kidneys, liver and lungs. Therefore, the lungs, which process oxygen and carbon dioxide (a by-product of cell metabolism), are critical to the removal of toxic waste, as they literally release or "blow off" acid and toxins from the body much like a catalytic converter and exhaust system in your car.

Blood serum levels can be assessed to determine if you are acid or alkaline, which indirectly reveals how you are doing with toxic removal and/or if you are accumulating too many toxins because of poor choices. Acid is constantly produced by cell function and increases when you are stressed. You may be aware (depending on your age) of what acid rain has done to cars; it causes a faster breakdown of metal. The world auto industry responded to this problem with sophisticated clear paint products to protect your investment. There is a blood test, called the anion gap, that indicates how your acid and alkaline system is responding. It helps a doctor see how your acid level is or is not handling the accelerated breakdown of your cells and body functions, including your blood vessels. Now, we all have some acid accumulation. How much, though, depends on your diet and stress levels; the more acid you have, the more quickly your cells will break down and not function at 100 percent. Since your body naturally gravitates to the acid side, you would do best to eat foods that create a more alkaline environment, which is why green veggies and select alkaline-producing fruits, like apples, are good for you; they help neutralize the acid. Please refer to the Page Diet found in Chapter 17.

I have found that when a patient finally gets the epiphany that it is time to modify the diet, when they start to eat "health" foods, which would include adding veggies and greens, they get nauseated—or just plain don't like them. The "repulsion" of green foods suggests to me that you are really acid and that your cells are being forced to dump toxic wastes and your system is not up to it. My suggestion is to begin by steaming, sautéing or lightly stir-frying veggies with olive or rice oils. This will cause the fiber to break down, making the vegetables easier to digest as well as helping your body adapt to the cleansing that is occurring at the cellular level.

I mentioned earlier a test called CRP, or C-reactive protein. There is an opinion that if this is elevated, you may have inflammation in your body, including in the walls of your blood vessels. I use this test with the anion gap and another test called the ESR (erythrocyte sedimentation rate) test to assess your state of inflammation. My experience, when correlating patient diet journals with test results, is that it's the men with fast food diets—loaded with grains, sodas and sugar—who have the most acid and inflammation.

When you are toxic, your body will retain fluid to hold the toxins in a state of solution so that they are less noxious while the liver, kidneys, skin and colon do their best to "dump" the debris. Therefore, another simple test I love to recommend, which you can do to yourself right now, is my very own "Dr. Bob's squeeze the wrist" test. While the test may not appear to be totally precise, it certainly is practical and does correlate to the results in the blood testing I assess with my patients. To begin, first look at your wrist: Do you see bone or a layer of "fat" or puffy tissue? Next, gently squeeze your wrist: Do you feel solid bone beneath or does it feel soft? What you do not want here is a squishy, boggy wrist, which, as I mentioned, is in direct response to the body accumulating extra fluid in order to dilute the toxins in a suspended solution of your own body fluids. Pass this process and information along to your friends.

If, when you perform the test, you do not feel a solid structure, evaluate what you have been consuming. Do you drink at least a quart of pure, clean water a day? Do you eat processed, "dead" foods or living, whole foods? Foods that are processed, packaged and lacking living nutrients tend to create a toxic state in your body. Once you change your diet—including cutting back to no sugar, trans fat or dairy products and adding cold-pressed olive, flax or marine oils—the fluid levels in your wrist will go down. You will see and feel your boney wrist once again and benefit from having far less of a burden from the accumulation of "extra" heart-straining fluids in your blood vessels. You are literally taking the proverbial monkey off your back, resulting in less heart stress and lower blood pressure, the importance of which we will discuss in this chapter.

BLOOD PRESSURE

Obesity is an issue impacting heart health because the heart is pumping the blood out of the largest blood vessel in the body, the aorta, and you do not want there to be any resistance. The blood vessel diameter, or the size of hole that blood travels through, decreases as the blood is delivered to the farthest parts of the body—the fingers and toes. When someone is overweight, the fat, or adipose tissue, in your body, which actually looks like yellow scrambled eggs, has to find areas to be released in, and since the blood vessels are hollow tubes, the fat cells compress down on them. With that compression, the heart has to beat extra hard to push the blood through. This creates an elevated resistance in the blood vessels with the probable result of high blood pressure. Other factors can then accentuate the resistance problem; a high-carbohydrate diet containing pastries, cookies, sodas and sweet fruits creates a normal body response of an increase in insulin, which then causes sodium retention, which then elevates fluid or water in the cardiovascular system. More water in smaller tubes can raise your blood pressure, just like a pump in your pond or backyard that is working really hard after a big rain. The low-fat, high-carbohydrate diet that many recommend today is the same type of diet the ancient Egyptians consumed. When the scientific community dissected the blood vessels of the ancient Egyptian mummies to assess blood vessel and cardiovascular integrity, they discovered scarring in the linings, a similar pattern found in autopsies today with high blood pressure issues, also seen on young men in the military.

I have mentioned sugar a few times as it relates to levels of inflammation in the body. Sugar is the real stealth saboteur. The typical American consumes the equivalent of one-half of a teaspoon of sugar every 30 minutes. Sugar is everywhere, it is becoming next to impossible to buy a product today that does not have some form of sugar in it, whether evaporated cane juice, sugar crystals, organic sugar, sugar, sucrose or high fructose corn syrup—the manufacturers attempt to hide the fact that there is sugar in the product. The real challenge with refined sugar is that it adds nothing to healthy body function, only calories. Sugar also depletes the body of critically needed minerals and vitamins, all of which are required for optimal cellular function. The immune system is paralyzed for hours when you eat a piece or two of cake or pie, a cookie, a pastry or ice cream. I commonly witness an increase of patients with chronic upper respiratory symptoms and sinus challenges on Mondays and following holidays where sugar and deserts were a focal point for celebrations. Sugar is addictive, a major cause of inflammation and pain and a leading cause of an acid state. Do you crave sugar? Sugar cravings can be cooled down with chromium supplementation. I have suggested up to nine tablets a day depending on the amount of sugar my patients are reporting in their diet journals that they have consumed. Saying NO to sugar is like saying NO to drugs. No exaggeration.

On top of a poor diet, many Americans suffer from the stress created by a hectic and overcommitted lifestyle. Stress compounds the problems with the heart; not only does it cause your body to become acid, but it can also elevate cortisol, which is secreted by the adrenal glands in times of emergency. With today's typically pressure-filled lifestyle, most people are in a low-grade level of emergency almost continuously, and this steady elevated cortisol level increases fluid retention and high blood pressure.

What You Can Do

Let's say you discover that your blood pressure is up, what should you do?

1. Lose weight.
2. Minimize your refined-carbohydrate, insulin-stimulating foods.

3. Evaluate your life circumstances and do what you can to minimize stress.

Should you take blood pressure–lowering medication? I would suggest that as the last resort. These medications trick your body. They create an imbalance in fluids and often will actually weaken heart muscle fibers. You may not die of a stroke or heart attack, but over time you will develop "flabby heart muscle" and succumb to congestive heart failure. Congestive heart failure is weakened heart tissue, and is often the result of years of taking medication.

Also, from my experience of over 35 years with this issue in patients, I do not recommend the use of commercial sodium chloride table salt, as it can create a mineral imbalance. I always advise using a full-spectrum mineral salt called Celtic Sea Salt®, which has magnesium, calcium and potassium to balance the sodium.

Understanding Blood Pressure Readings

Let's now look at the two numbers you see in your blood pressure readings and their significance in your long-term health strategy. The top number is called the systolic pressure. This is the amount of pressure your lower heart, or ventricles, push to get the blood to the distal, or faraway, parts of the body. The lower number is called the diastolic pressure. The diastolic reading is affected by the amount of pressure that is placed on the blood vessels as they are returning blood to the heart. The normal blood pressure numbers are 120 over 80, written as 120/80. When the top number is over, let's say, 140, it can be for a number of reasons. For example, the systolic level will go up if you are overweight, as discussed. When the diastolic pressure is elevated, let's say, above 90, you have the potential of having heart muscle stress.

Contrary to what you will hear in the media, I have found in my practice, and have likewise seen reported by Donald LePore, ND, in his book The Ultimate Healing System, that the systolic pressure (top number) can be improved with sodium and the diastolic pressure (bottom number) can be controlled with potassium. The one food that has a natural balance of sodium and potassium is alfalfa. I have witnessed blood pressure return to normal with up to nine alfalfa tablets a day. I have also observed the same results with kelp tablet supplementation up to nine a day and have had excellent patient results, as mentioned above, using Celtic Sea Salt®.

That brings us to an important point about salt I'd like to clarify. Americans are warned against consuming too much sodium, and most do consume too much from sources like fast and convenience foods. The salt in those foods is highly unhealthy because it is not balanced by minerals. Therefore, I encourage my patients to get their sodium from whole, balanced sodium from Celtic Sea Salt®, celery and beets. I consistently see great outcomes with this plan. For more information on this subject, see Dr. David Brownstein's book Salt Your Way to Health, in which he discusses his research into the use of quality unrefined salt.

One other thought I'd like to share about blood pressure issues and normal readings: Proper positioning or alignment of the upper vertebra in the spine by a skilled chiropractor can lower a person's blood pressure up to 17 points. It takes two blood pressure pills to create the same results! The spinal correction is a safe and effective way to help assist the body to heal itself. I have repeatedly seen this occur since 1978.

HOW THYROID FUNCTION IMPACTS THE HEART

A subpar or poor thyroid function has a potentially negative impact on heart health due to its effect on cholesterol metabolism and another item called homocysteine. In a nutshell, when the thyroid is stuck on low, LDL ("bad"—but not really; you will learn more about this later in the chapter) cholesterol tends to elevate, with or without dietary restrictions. Your goal should be to have your LDL cholesterol below 75 as a way to prevent potential atherosclerosis or fat in the lining of the blood vessels. I have witnessed elevated LDL cholesterol levels in patients who eat what I call an inflammation diet, which is one that is full of snack and convenience foods loaded with trans fat. Even the "heart healthy" breakfast cereal with the "stealth" trans fat disguised by the scientific name "partially hydrogenated" fat, which is actually trans fat, is a part of this diet! You would not think the mid-morning pastry, donuts at meetings or fried foods easily picked up at the drive-thru are causing elevated levels of inflammation in your unsuspecting blood vessels. Few of my patients have previously correlated food with inflammation.

Over the past decade, research has identified another factor that seems to be as important as diet and lifestyle in creating heart disease. That risk factor is high blood levels of the amino acid homocysteine. Homocysteine is created when another amino acid, methionine—found in red meat, milk and milk products—is broken down in the body. Under ideal circumstances, the body breaks down homocysteine with the help of vitamins B6, B12 and folic acid.

Studies continue to establish stronger links between even moderately elevated blood levels of homocysteine and heart disease. In the 1992 Physicians' Health Study, men with very high homocysteine levels had a risk of heart attack three times that of men with normal homocysteine levels. In fact, an elevated homocysteine level was such a dominant factor that it indicated increased risk even in the men who had no other cardiovascular risks.

Because of the importance of homocysteine levels as a heart attack risk factor, efforts have thus far concentrated on lowering high levels through any means possible. And up until now, the only consistently successful approach has been to increase the intake of whole-food B vitamins. However, new research indicates that lowering homocysteine levels in this manner may be simply masking a more serious underlying problem that causes the elevation in the first place. The bigger problem is an underactive thyroid.

Researchers at the Cleveland Clinic have released findings showing that correcting an underactive thyroid gland normalizes elevated homocysteine levels in the blood. Even more amazing is that the researchers were able to normalize homocysteine levels without having to administer any of the B vitamins. In other words, correcting the thyroid condition in turn corrected the vitamin deficiency.[1] Iodine is one of the key "players" for optimal thyroid function and therefore very important for heart health. According to the World Health Organization, up to 72 percent of the world's population does not get enough iodine in their diets. We will discuss the thyroid in detail later in the book.

IMPROVING HEART HEALTH

When it comes to improving heart health, we are dealing with several issues:

1. Creating unrestricted movement of blood (flawless blood flow)
2. Strengthening heart tissue
3. Reducing whatever is causing the inflammation in the vessels
4. Normalizing thyroid function
5. Assessing homocysteine levels and correcting accordingly

Did you know that flaxseed oil, rich in omega-3 fat, when taken regularly promotes a healthy environment with the production of long-chain fatty acids (eicosapentaenoic acid, or EPA for short) and a fat tissue hormone called prostaglandin 3, or PG3, minimizes inflammation? If you start eating walnuts, mixed greens, green beans and flax oil, you'll be moving in a good direction. Salmon is also excellent, but you need to be doubly sure that it is coming from the ocean and that you are not purchasing the farm-raised variety. Unfortunately, today you have to be careful because seafood may have contaminants in the flesh and fat, where toxins are stored. I recommend never eating farm-raised fish because of the contaminants they get from the antibiotics and food-coloring pellets that are added to their food. Whatever the fish eats, you absorb. I was recently advised that some companies that process "marine oil"—oil sourced from ocean fish, which would include salmon, tuna, cod and others—were allowing toxic levels of harmful chemicals in the content of their capsules, and I have also heard that some manufacturers may, in fact, have capsules that are not safe. The toxins in the oil are unfortunately from chemicals from the ocean, which in many places has become highly polluted. I actually only eat fish given to me from a patient who travels to northern Canada and catches them from a lake that does not have industrial or farm runoff.

The marine-sourced oil I use is sourced from anchovy and sardine oils. Because these types of fish do not have much fat, toxins generally do not accumulate in them. I do want you to be aware, too, that taking any marine oil, including salmon oil that is liquid or in capsule form, can thin your blood too much; so I do not recommend regular usage of these if you live in a temperate climate. People in northern, cold climates like Alaska and northern Canada have a metabolism that utilizes oils at a different level. In my practice, I test my patients' current blood fat levels with a blood spot test and then recommend a strategy of exact oils to normalize their fat metabolism. I have found that most of my patients are better served if they use a plant-sourced omega-3 fat like flax or black currant seed oil. I discuss this and cholesterol at great length in my book *Dr. Bob's Trans Fat Survival Guide.*

OTHER SIGNS OF HEART DISTRESS

Another interesting correlation I have discovered over time is that your body type can also help determine if you may be a candidate for heart challenges. There is one particular body type common in men, though both genders can have it, where the abdomen is quite large and protruding. It is this body type where heart problems are most likely to occur. Large abdomens usually suggest a congested liver. The blood in your body naturally flows from the distal, or far-away, parts on its way back to the heart. The blood travels through the liver to be processed and filtered. And here is the crucial point I have consistently observed: A congested liver can impede or slow the blood flow on the way back to the heart.

I have an instrument called an acoustic cardiogram, which is an electronic stethoscope that senses sounds and translates them from vibrations to a graph, or mechanical energy. The stethoscope is placed over four different areas or valve regions of the heart. Each acoustic placement evaluation on the chest wall creates a different perspective of how the heart functions. The noise or sounds are created by the valves closing. The valves are affected by the heart muscle that is creating the motion closing the valves. When the blood flow is impeded by the slowing of the flow through the liver on the way back to the heart, it shows up on the graph as a round elevation rather than a sharp spike.

I also notice patterns of nearly constant pyramid-shaped, high and low zigzagging lines instead of a flat line graph. These correspond to the inconsistent opening and closing of valves, represented on the graph as a pattern of static waves. When I review the diet journals of these patients, I find that they are persistent wheat eaters. Wheat and other grains such as rye, oats and spelt have gluten in their makeup. Gluten does what it sounds like: It literally will glue the little villi or projections in the intestines that absorb minerals, preventing them from taking in critically needed nutrients. Wheat eaters can also have inflammation, as revealed on the Adrenal Gland Stress Saliva Index (ASI) tests I complete on my patients. Wheat, therefore, may be a component of your heart distress. Think about how many pastries, sandwiches and pizzas you eat. The reality may alarm you! If you want to help your heart, try going gluten free for a month and see what happens to your chest tightness, leg cramps and energy. You will be pleasantly amazed!

Other signs of heart trouble reveal themselves to the aware observer. You can obviously tell by looking at patients which ones are overweight. But there are also those who have a history of gallbladder surgery, and I learn this from my intake form when patients first come to see me. When someone has their gallbladder removed, their liver has not been functioning optimally, and this, as just discussed, can affect the heart. The liver operates similarly to the oil filter in your car, which you know from the owner's manual needs to be replaced in a timely fashion or the engine will malfunction. Just as dirty driving conditions will clog your filter more quickly than a cleaner environment would, you literally clog your liver with the fried foods you eat, the milkshakes and alcohol you drink and the medicines you take to treat the symptoms of not taking care of yourself. By the way, you also add the right oil to the engine of your car for top performance, just like I am recommending that you "add" the right oil to your body's "engine"!

I also observe my patients' ear lobes, as those who have a history of heart distress appear to have a small crease on the lobe. This is an acupuncture point associated with heart physiology. With acupuncture, we are able to affect the flow of energy by placing delicate needles into certain points in the body. Interestingly, placing pierced ear rings in the lobe actually has the potential to stimulate optimal heart function. This may be a thought to consider nowadays, since more men are having their ears pierced in the lobe.

SHOULD YOU TAKE
CHOLESTEROL-LOWERING DRUGS?

What about some of the medications you have read about for lowering cholesterol? Should you take them? The best known drugs in this category are the statins, so let's discuss those first. One problem with statin drugs is they create liver distress. In fact, the negative effects of statin drugs can be devastating. I have heard all the radio ads on statins suggesting that they can lower your cholesterol up to 39 percent. Well, did you know that beets, consumed cooked or raw, can lower your cholesterol just as much, if not more? Yes, you read that right—beets! Dr. Gina Nick, in her book Clinical Purification, stated that it has been clinically proven that you can lower your cholesterol up to 40 percent by adding beet fiber, 15 grams a few times a week, to your diet. I personally eat up to a half a beet daily on my mixed green power salad at lunch. The reason this simple root works is that cholesterol attaches itself to the beet fiber and is released through the colon. Oatmeal has similar properties, so if you like oatmeal for breakfast, eat the "gluten free" variety.

To get this benefit from beets you can bake, steam or pressure-cook them. Do not boil them. Do not eat canned or pickled beets. Here's a quick recipe: Cut the beets in slices about ½" to ¾" thick. Put a small amount of water in the bottom of your baking dish. Bake the beets at 400° Fahrenheit for one hour or so. Cover and check with a fork for tenderness. Let them cool, or eat them with olive or flax oil. The only side effect of this amazing cholesterol-lowering treatment is that your stool (bowel movement) or urine may be red. This is not harmful.

There are cholesterol-lowering medications that interrupt cholesterol absorption in the intestines, and there are other meds that are combinations of colon fat cholesterol "soppers" and statin liver meds. In studies, both have been shown to not lower cholesterol safely or, in some cases, not without very serious side effects—optic stroke, liver disease, muscle pain syndrome, erectile dysfunction, lowered levels of coenzyme Q10 needed for optimal heart function, and fatty acid mal-absorption syndromes. Because of the side effects and danger of these medications, I suggest your long-term strategy for longevity and heart protection include your determination to avoid the foods that cause inflammation in the first place—sugar, dairy, ice cream, yogurt and wheat. You are already watching the beef, right?

I encourage my patients to minimize refined sugar and avoid sugar substitutes, including sucralose and aspartame, as you go through your transition from good to better to best. We'll talk more about natural, healthy alternatives later. You might not like beets—I understand. Frankly, I didn't care for Brussels sprouts until I started eating real fresh ones and sautéing them with mushrooms and onions. But if someone suggested a natural and healthy food choice that would minimize another medication that has severe side effects, I would eat it until I eliminated the cause of my problem. And again, not to be redundant, the root of the problem is inflammation caused by refined sugar, of which the average American eats an alarming amount—around 150 pounds per year—and trans fat, which was actually once thought to be a heart hero.

VITAMIN D AND HEART HEALTH

You may not have thought about it, but vitamin D has a role in heart health. Vitamin D, which, by the way, is not actually a vitamin but is rather a pro-hormone (a precursor to a hormone), impacts the utilization of calcium in the body. Calcium helps calm the whole system, including blood pressure and vessel walls. Vitamin D creates the withdrawal of calcium from the intestines into the blood. Therefore, it is important that you take calcium when taking vitamin D. I recommend taking a vitamin D test to get a basis of where your levels are, especially if you or your family has a history of heart distress. If your skin itches when you take vitamin D, it may mean that you do not have enough calcium in your tissues. I recommend anywhere from 1,200 to 1,400 mg of calcium lactate or citrate a day, to be taken on an empty stomach. Omega-3 oils like flax oil help the transfer of calcium from the blood to the skin. Additionally, you should have at least one-half the amount of magnesium compared to calcium, so at least 600 mg a day. I generally recommend adults take 2,000 IU of vitamin D a day, and even up to 10,000 IU. Children can take anywhere from 800 to 2,000 IU of vitamin D daily.

Cholecalciferol, also called vitamin D3, is the most beneficial form of vitamin D for health. Sunshine exposure is the most efficient and best way to achieve optimal vitamin D3 levels. Sunshine converts the cholesterol in your skin to vitamin D through a series of metabolic pathways that also include the liver and kidney. You can consume vitamin D from food, but I have noticed when I assess patients' vitamin D levels, those who work in the sun have higher vitamin D levels than those who work in an office or with little natural sun exposure. Also, people living in the northern areas above the year-round sunshine line will get less D than those exposed to sunlight more often. The best time to have the right sunrays on your skin is before 11 a.m. and then between 4 p.m. and 6 p.m., with 85 percent of your body exposed. Avoid the most damaging rays of the sun that occur between 11 a.m. and 3 p.m. Suntan lotion prevents the cholesterol in your skin from being metabolized to vitamin D. That's why it's important to get rays during the least damaging times of day, when you can safely be exposed without needing sunblock to protect your skin.

I have found that in snowbirds from the north visiting sunny regions during the winter, exposure to the sun will keep the vitamin D levels within normal for up to a month after returning to the sunless north. These folks may want to add vitamin D when they get home for a month or so before they have their natural vitamin D sourced from the sun.

Individuals with dark skin tend to have lower levels of vitamin D when I test them. I have yet to have one dark-skinned patient have a level above 20, when 40 is normal. Therefore, I encourage all of my dark-skinned patients to have their vitamin D tested.

Given this range of dynamics, it may be easier and more effective to take a D supplement to control vitamin D levels. For this, I do not recommend synthetic D2, which nearly all the prescription-based supplements contain. Instead, go for cod liver oil or even whole eggs (including the yolk). Farm-raised fish does not give the amount of D that ocean fish provides. Because of the limited non-vegan sources of vitamin D, vegetarians tend to have a deficiency of it. If you're a vegetarian and are opposed to eating eggs or taking fish oil, then there are vitamin D3 supplements on the market made from olive and coconut oils. Whatever your D supplement preference is, be sure to get out and get at least a little sun as well.

Blood pressure levels will lower and stabilize with proper vitamin D supplementation. I generally recommend 2,000 IU daily as a minimum but have some patients take up to 50,000 IUs until their serum levels increase to normal. I have had many patients lower their blood pressure to normal just by supplementing their D levels after they discovered how low in D they were—one patient's level was 9, when, as I mentioned, normal is 40.

TYPES OF HEART MALFUNCTION

Following are some of the most common heart-related problems and issues surrounding them. There are many types of conditions that impact the heart. Historically men tend to have more heart challenges than women, partially because of physical makeup along with personal and financial responsibility, which of course is changing as women are now being impacted by role reversals. I have listed some common challenges that I consult and treat in my practice.

Angina

Angina is chest pain or discomfort that happens when the heart does not get enough blood. It may feel like a pressing or squeezing pain, often in the chest, but sometimes the pain is in the shoulders, arms, neck, jaw or back. It can also feel like indigestion (upset stomach). Angina is not a heart attack.

Heart Attack

A heart attack occurs when an artery is severely or completely blocked, which can occur for a number of reasons—including clot; inflammation; narrowing; and thick, fat blood from eating refined foods—and therefore the heart tissue does not get the blood it needs for more than 20 minutes. Young individuals have a greater chance of dying from a heart attack because, unlike older patients, who have anastomoses or the growth of finger-like projections of small vessels with new blood flow, they are not capable of withstanding a large reduction of blood flow. Older patients have a new source of oxygen from these new growths. Commonly the first symptom in a heart attack for those under 40 tends to be the last one; rarely do younger victims get a second chance. I'm explaining this for you men who are between 25 and 40 who think you are excused to eat and carry on with reckless abandon—this is serious. I recently had an acquaintance who was the guest musician at an event I was attending die suddenly of a heart attack the week after we returned home. I had mentioned to my wife at the event that the man had "put on a bit of weight." He was 40 when he died, leaving several young children to face life without a father. At the wake, his daughter made light of the fact that her dad had a passionate addiction to a "fancy named" high-end coffee drink with 750 calories per drink …Gentlemen, I repeat, this is serious! Do you have enough life insurance?

Heart Failure

Heart failure occurs when the heart is not able to pump blood through the body as well as it should. This means that other organs, which normally get blood from the heart, do not get enough blood. It does not mean that the heart stops. I see this in patients who have been on blood pressure medication and diuretics for long-term usage. Signs of heart failure include:

- Shortness of breath (feeling like you can't get enough air)
- Swelling in feet, ankles and legs
- Extreme tiredness

Heart Arrhythmias

These are changes in the beat of the heart. Most people have felt dizzy, faint, out of breath or had chest pains at one time or another. These changes in heartbeat are, for most people, harmless. As you get older, you are more likely to have arrhythmias. Don't panic if you have a few flutters or if your heart races once in a while. The flutters and other symptoms such as dizziness or shortness of breath may be a deficiency of whole-food B vitamins.

HEART HEALTH FACTS FOR OPTIMAL FUNCTION

There are many facets of heart health. Anytime you pick up a magazine or search the Internet, it seems like there is an article about something new you can add to your daily routine that will restore heart function. We will talk about some of the most beneficial suggestions below, as well as about certain products that, although promoted as heart healthy, are, in fact, just the opposite.

Antioxidants

Antioxidants such as vitamins C and E operate to protect your cells against the effects of free radicals, which are potentially damaging by-products of energy metabolism. Free radicals can damage cells and may contribute to the development of cardiovascular disease and cancer. Vitamins C and E have the ability to limit production of free radicals, and thus might help prevent or delay the development of those chronic diseases. Vitamins C and E have also been shown to play a role in immune function, DNA repair and other metabolic processes.

To get the full power and benefit from vitamins C and E, you need to get them from a whole-food source rather than synthetic. I have found that a great source of antioxidants, minerals and other life-enhancing nutrients is the apple. I encourage all of my patients to eat half an apple every single day. Red apples are especially recommended, as green apples tend to cause digestion to stagnate. Other foods with vitamins C and E that provide antioxidant protection include organic pressed vegetable oils, nuts, green leafy vegetables and whole grain cereals. A great simple source of healthy snack food and fiber also would include red, yellow and orange bell peppers.

LDL and HDL

While there is a lot of discussion about "good" versus "bad" cholesterol, I actually don't think of cholesterol in those terms—but rather only as necessary for survival. Cholesterol acts as a type of firefighter in the body, being transported to any site that needs it for the purpose of "extinguishing" inflammation. Since it is not water soluble, it cannot dissolve in the blood and has to be transported to and from cells by carriers called lipoproteins. Low-density lipoprotein, or LDL, has been labeled as "bad" cholesterol. High-density lipoprotein, or HDL, is known as "good" cholesterol. These two types of lipids, along with triglycerides (discussed in a moment) and cholesterol, make up your total cholesterol count, which can be determined through a blood test.

When you are consuming food that creates inflammation, more LDL will be transported to minimize the inflammation. When too much LDL "bad" (but not really, as it is going to the fire) cholesterol circulates in the blood, it can slowly build up in the inner walls of the arteries that feed the heart and brain. Together with other substances, it can form plaque—a thick, hard deposit that can narrow the arteries and make them less flexible—resulting in the condition known as atherosclerosis. If a clot forms and blocks a narrowed artery, a heart attack or stroke can result. This is, of course, the reason LDL gets such a bad rap. However, the body is doing what it can to protect itself. The truly important question, which is rarely asked, is "What is causing the fire?" The answer is the usual culprits: sugar, dairy and trans fat, which we will continue to discuss throughout the rest of this book.

About one-fourth to one-third of blood cholesterol is carried by high-density lipoprotein (HDL). The reason why HDL cholesterol is known as "good" cholesterol is that high levels of HDL seem to protect against heart attack. Conversely, low levels of HDL (less than 40 mg/dL) increase the risk of heart disease. HDL carries cholesterol away from the arteries and back to the liver, where it's passed from the body. Some experts believe that HDL removes excess cholesterol from arterial plaque, slowing its buildup. In my practice, I have been able to help increase patients' HDL levels with chromium and phosphatidylcholine supplementation.

As a side note here, if you're a senior citizen, you don't want your cholesterol count to be lower than 200, regardless of what you've been told. When cholesterol is lower than 160, with or without medication, you may have challenges with cancer and memory issues.

Triglycerides

Triglyceride is a form of fat made in the body. Elevated triglycerides can be due to excess weight/obesity, physical inactivity, cigarette smoking and excess alcohol consumption. Additionally, a diet very high in refined carbohydrates, meaning that 60 percent or more of total calories are derived from sugary carbs, such as pastas, cookies, pastries, potato chips, breads and sweet fruits—yes, sweet fruits like bananas, pineapple and dried fruits can elevate triglycerides. People with high triglycerides often have a high total cholesterol level, including a high LDL level and a low HDL level. Many people with heart disease and/or diabetes also have high triglyceride levels. Diabetics have increased blood fats because of poor metabolism of the carbohydrates they are consuming.

Aspirin

Are you taking an aspirin a day? How much are you taking? How do you know that what you're taking is the right amount? Do you understand why you are taking the aspirin? While many people follow their doctor's advice for a baby aspirin a day to prevent heart attack by thinning the blood and making blood cells less "sticky," they are completely unaware that taking any amount of aspirin without being monitored is like playing Russian roulette. It just isn't safe. For example, did you know that consistent aspirin indulgence can create ulcers, digestive distress and even stroke? Or that long-term aspirin usage can result in liver disease?

It may take time, but I can promise you that over months and years you may begin noticing easy bruising on your skin, a pit in your stomach and even a black tar substance in the toilet (this last one is a signal that your stomach may be bleeding). These negative effects are the result of your blood cells becoming fragile and easily broken. Aspirin usage can even slow down the healing of bones. If it can do this, then, is it a leap to think that it may also create the environment that precipitates osteoporosis?

Despite these serious drawbacks, I am not suggesting that you stop taking aspirin without first talking to your health care provider. I educate and diligently work with my patients by having their essential fats or essential fatty acids (EFAs) tested, which we will discuss in detail in Chapter 4. The EFA blood spot test shows exactly which fatty acids are in excess and which are deficient in your body. One of the side effects of aspirin, which is thought to be a benefit for heart health, is that it stops or diminishes the formation of the fat-like tissue hormone prostaglandin 2, or PG2, which causes red blood cells to stick together, hardens blood vessels and increases pain. The aspirin is tricking the body by sabotaging PG2 production. What is actually going on with conventional medicine in our society today is the treatment of symptoms with procedures that work from the outside in—such as taking an aspirin without a thought about the real cause of the problem—eating food that causes blood cells to stick together.

The Real Cause of the "Silent Killer"

High blood pressure is often referred to as the "silent killer" because people with high blood pressure often have no symptoms and can die without warning. In my experience, the real cause behind high blood pressure is the sequence and crescendo of adrenal gland distress, exhaustion and finally fatigue. As discussed in Chapter 1, the adrenal glands are located on top of the kidneys and have many functions, including controlling mineral movement in the body and stabilizing blood sugar with the release of cortisol. The adrenal glands secrete hormones that speed the body up, getting ready for a burst of energy to help you escape a harmful situation. Our human bodies were designed to respond to emergencies with enormous capabilities to move us out of harm's way. Well, today, there is constant stimulation to the adrenal glands, with small, continuous alarms firing all the time. The resulting ever-persistent release of stress hormones puts the body on alert, constantly ready to go, yet there is no real danger, only stimulation and a state of readiness!

When your adrenal glands are distressed, your heart is affected. This is the reason some people are put on meds to block the impact of the stress hormones on the heart. The adrenal glands are responding to stimuli either apparent physically or mentally in the form of worry and/or anxiety. Hormones are released by the adrenals for the body to respond, including a demand placed on the heart to "get going." The constant barrage of stimuli to the heart and vessels results in your heart being on a constant ever-ready alert; your blood pressure is up. Beta blocker medications are a common medical protocol prescribed to control or lower blood pressure. In essence, you are confusing the system with meds that create more of a challenge with their side effects, including erectile dysfunction in men.

One way to get your adrenal glands in better working order is to get enough rest. Your body needs to sleep, as this is when growth hormone is produced. While you are sleeping, growth hormone is released by your brain to repair your body, much like the way maintenance work is completed on delivery vehicles while they are being loaded in the warehouse—during downtime. Rest precludes restoration and is critical for optimal health. You should wake up well rested and hungry in the morning. If you are having trouble sleeping, I suggest avoiding the stimulation of watching television or using the computer before going to bed, as this has been shown to make falling asleep more difficult. I would not get addicted to sleeping aids. I have found that when the adrenal glands are rested, your sleep will naturally be restored.

Regarding adrenal gland function, low blood pressure can be as unhealthy as high blood pressure is. As the heart continues to pump blood to nourish tissues, the adrenal glands are partially responsible for your blood pressure level by, as mentioned earlier, releasing hormones that speed the heart up or slow it down. When your body is in a constant state of alert and the adrenal glands are forced to respond, over time they literally become exhausted and stop working to their full capacity. An example of how your body may be handling stress can be measured by the amount of pain you are in and what you need to do to eliminate the pain. If you are taking or have been prescribed a treatment that uses cortisone or something derived from steroids and you feel great while you are on the program or had the injection, but as time goes on and the effect of the medication is over and the pain once again returns, your adrenal glands are more than likely exhausted.

One of the findings of adrenal gland exhaustion is low blood pressure or a blood pressure level that drops when switching from a sitting to a standing position. Your blood pressure may, for example, be 130/80, but when you stand up it may drop to 115/70 or even lower. With results like this, I would suspect that your adrenal function is being compromised either from stress or from you eating too much sugar. When these factors are present, your adrenal glands have to work harder and harder to make sure your pressure stays high enough for your heart to have some blood to push through the system. Low blood pressure is very common in my patients who are near physical and mental exhaustion.

To raise low blood pressure to an acceptable range and for heart health, I suggest herbal supplements such as licorice root or Rehmannia (an adrenal gland adaptogen) and a whole-food B vitamin. To lower your blood pressure, I recommend minimizing sugar, drinking more water and using Celtic Sea Salt®. Minerals are important for the body; today many people's bodies are screaming for more of them. What you eat has an important effect on your mineral level. For instance, wheat bread and products with soy deplete zinc in the body. On the other hand, using Celtic Sea Salt® daily helps replace critical minerals. In fact, drinking water with a quarter teaspoon of Celtic Sea Salt® will give your body much-needed minerals. B vitamins will also help if you are experiencing heart palpitations or a "racing heart." Exercising also contributes to a healthy heart, but don't overdo it. Your body needs a balance of exercise and rest.

ATTACK HEART ATTACKS AND HIGH BLOOD PRESSURE – ACTION STEPS

☐ **Know your blood pressure:** Your heart moves blood through your body. If it is hard for your heart to do this, your heart works harder and your blood pressure will rise. Years of high blood pressure can lead to heart disease and failure. Since people with high blood pressure often have no symptoms, have your blood pressure checked every six months and make the required lifestyle changes: lose weight, exercise and minimize stress. Take heart medication as a last resort.

☐ **Have testing done:** You may want to have your thyroid tested, and we'll discuss this more in Chapter 8. Low thyroid is associated with high homocysteine levels. Your homocysteine and vitamin D levels would be good to know since homocysteine levels elevate with potential heart disease whereas vitamin D levels may be low. CRP levels may be elevated with inflammation.

☐ **Don't smoke:** If you smoke, quit. If you're having trouble quitting, there are natural products and programs that can help:

   ✓ Nicotine Relief®, a proprietary product from GAIA Herbs, is helpful for stopping the tobacco cravings. It can be found on my website (**www.druglessdoctor.com**) or wherever the product line is sold.

   ✓ Niacinamide: 500 to 1,000 mg a day. This helps create the nicotinic acid the brain and body is craving in cigarettes.

✓ Royal Jelly: up to 2,000 mg a day. This bee product assists the body not to crave tobacco.

✓ Lobelia, an herb that reduces anxiety associated with cigarette cravings

✓ Create new patterns of daily activity where you do not smoke. For example, go to work using a different route, do not smoke with coffee, eat celery (celery helps having something in your mouth, and actually requires more calories to process than it adds, so you won't gain weight; I buy celery hearts), and so on.

☐ **Eat whole foods:** Avoid sugar, dairy and trans fat. Do not buy "0 grams trans fat" products without first looking at the ingredients to see if there is partially hydrogenated oils in the list, as this is just another name for trans fat. And no ice cream or yogurt—they are usually high in sugar.

☐ **Maintain a healthy weight:** Being overweight raises your risk for heart disease. Eat a healthy diet, and exercise at a moderate intensity for at least 30 minutes every day. Add more vegetables and whole grains, but avoid wheat products in your diet. Take a brisk walk daily or take the stairs instead of the elevator. Focus on mid-glycemic-index foods that do not create sugar cravings and increase insulin. Elevated insulin levels promote fat storage versus fat burning; therefore, avoid refined grain foods and pastries.

☐ **Eliminate alcohol, including wine:** Alcohol creates stress on the liver, promoting accelerated death. Though wine is promoted as a heart tonic, from my experience drinking wine is not going to produce long-term heart health. Despite its other properties, wine still has a percentage of alcohol in its ingredients, and alcohol needs to be processed by the liver. And, as you've learned, liver health is critical for heart health. Alcohol can also create an increased appetite, which means you will eat more and gain more weight, further compounding your heart issues.

☐ **Find healthy ways to cope with stress:** Lower your stress level by learning to say, "No." Stop doing everything you are asked to do. It is time for a rest. Make yours and your family's health a priority. The adrenals will continue to release the hormones to speed the body up unless "YOU" decide to give it a rest—give your heart a break.

4

FACTS ABOUT FAT

This chapter is, by far, one of the most important pieces of information you will ever read. I promise it will be really simple. Let me set the tone. I treat patients, naturally, every day. I am not force-fed information by pharmaceutical detail men. I study the results I see with my patients and use them to create more effective treatment protocols. Regardless of who you are, physiology is physiology. Water freezes at 32° Fahrenheit no matter what a person's health care background is. The word "doctor" comes from the Latin verb *docere*, which means "to teach." My intent here is not to impress you with big words, formulas or jargon, but rather to teach you about fat and its effects on your health. I am going to relay to you what I have seen in over 30 years in my practice. This is not a blind study, or money-driven or hypothetical information; it is observations of results, victories and setbacks from real people, the people who wake up in the morning hungry, have kids to feed, groceries to buy, schedules to keep and lifestyles to maintain.

Not too long ago I had a discussion with a friend about health. He lifts weights, exercises aerobically, sees natural doctors and, generally, from the outside, appears to be in excellent shape for his chronological age. I asked him the same question I am going to ask you: "Do you know what trans fat is?" A glassy, blank stare with a statue-like facial expression appeared as he said, "I do not have a clue what you're talking about." I asked if he was sure. Embarrassingly and not wanting to hurt my feelings, he responded, "No, and probably very few other people I know do either." End of conversation.

The very next day, I was scheduled to speak to a group of over 130 people about ADHD, Alzheimer's and depression. This was to be a mixed-age group, with attendees from various cultural and socio-economic backgrounds. *WOW!* I thought, *I'll ask them the same question I posed to my friend.* At the event, I explained to them about my research for the book I was writing at the time, *Dr. Bob's Trans Fat Survival Guide,* and wanted a show of hands as to how many knew what trans fat was. Only 10 people raised their hands. I was taken aback. It occurred to me that we are truly experiencing the same mindset that people had centuries ago concerning scurvy. No one knew that a lack of vitamin C was killing their families, just as these individuals did not realize that trans fat is *the* leading factor for ADHD, Alzheimer's and depression. All of these conditions are in an epidemic growth pattern and no one seems to understand why. Now for the rest of the story.

For some people, such as my fitness trainer's husband, who never ever eats any type of fat or food with fat in it, the mere thought of fat passing through their lips can create convulsive gyrations. But fat is important. It gives taste to food, and your body needs fat to function. This is sometimes a surprise to people. Your body uses fat for fuel, insulation, to make hormones and to send messages along cell membranes. It is also used to isolate toxins and provide a protective coating in blood vessels to keep them from damage and to relieve pain.

My first easy-to-understand discussion here is about a fat classification called essential fats or essential fatty acids (EFAs). You see, the mass confusion about fats lies in all the classifications and possibilities. But this will be easy-easy-easy, I promise. There are only two essential fats. They are termed "essential" because the body doesn't produce them; to get them, you need to eat them. If you don't eat them, you can't use them. These fats are used by the body to make other fats that are essential for life. My own study on this topic points to a lack of quality-sourced essential fats as the primary cause of our modern health problems. So, being such an important matter, let's start by looking at the first of the two essential fats or EFAs.

LINOLEIC ACID

The first essential fat is linoleic acid, which is pronounced the way it looks: "lynn-o-lay-ik." This fat is commonly found in foods and can be in oil form as well. For example, natural sources for linoleic acid include most seeds and nuts, plus safflower and sunflower oils. These food items and oils can be considered "precursors." That means that the linoleic fats you eat need to go through steps to become other important factors your body needs. These steps require vitamins and minerals such as calcium, magnesium, zinc, vitamin B and vitamin B6 (see Chart #1).

Deficiencies, then, in any of these vitamins and minerals can interrupt your body's ability to build and repair itself. The body is a self-healing organism. Certain enzymes are also part of the process. These enzymes and vitamins can become deficient from poor absorption that occurs because of the aging process or from medication that impairs nutrient absorption. Reread this paragraph and get ready. What I am going to say next is BIG.

The process for linoleic acid continues on to become a final item called prostaglandin 1, or PG1. Prostaglandins are fat, tissue-like hormones that are necessary *for critical life-enhancing functions*. PG1 takes away pain and makes blood cells less sticky and vessel walls more pliable. Simply put, PG1 is heart healthy and pain relieving.

There are multiple enzymes and nutrients, including vitamins and minerals, needed to complete the process of creating PG1. An

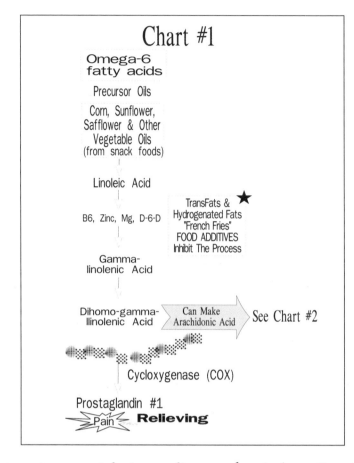

Chart #1

Omega-6 fatty acids

Precursor Oils

Corn, Sunflower, Safflower & Other Vegetable Oils (from snack foods)

Linoleic Acid

B6, Zinc, Mg, D-6-D

TransFats & Hydrogenated Fats "French Fries" FOOD ADDITIVES Inhibit The Process

Gamma-linolenic Acid

Dihomo-gamma-llinolenic Acid — Can Make Arachidonic Acid — See Chart #2

Cycloxygenase (COX)

Prostaglandin #1
Pain Relieving

enzyme acts as a catalyst, speeding up chemical reactions inside living things. In the case of the process we are discussing, you can think of an enzyme like a little freight ship moving cargo in and out of harbor. One enzyme, called cyclooxygenase (see Chart #2), has been the target of modern pain-relieving pharmaceutical research teams. Commonly called a COX inhibitor, it is the family of enzymes targeted by Vioxx® and Celebrex® in the formation of prostaglandin 2, or PG2, which creates pain and causes blood cells to stick. When these enzymes are targeted by a drug for one function, the ripple effect creates physiologic havoc elsewhere. You will read more about COX inhibitors in Chapter 5. But I'm getting ahead of myself with PG2. Let's back up a bit.

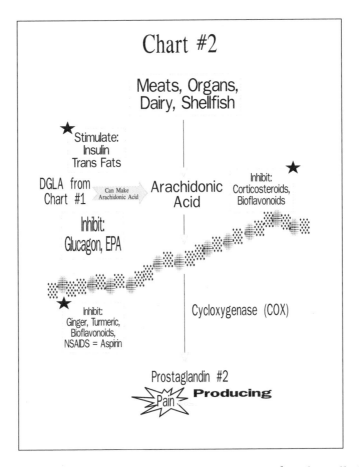

Chart #2

Meats, Organs,
Dairy, Shellfish

★ Stimulate:
Insulin
Trans Fats

DGLA from   Can Make   Arachidonic   Inhibit:
Chart #1   Arachidonic Acid   Acid   Corticosteroids, ★
                                        Bioflavonoids

Inhibit:
Glucagon, EPA

★ Inhibit:
Ginger, Turmeric,
Bioflavonoids,
NSAIDS = Aspirin

Cycloxygenase (COX)

Prostaglandin #2
Pain Producing

In its passage, linoleic acid can also become another fat called arachidonic acid. Arachidonic acid can become PG2. PG2 is necessary so you feel pain and don't bleed to death, and therefore, helps you get the message that you need rest and healing. The interim step to creating arachidonic acid is displayed in Chart #2. The fat here is called dihomogamma-linolenic acid, or DGLA. Your body, in its ability to self-regulate, needs to increase the formation of arachidonic acid for the balance of other fats. The creation of arachidonic acid is one of the reasons some scientists believe we need to eat less food, fat and oil with linoleic acid features. We get too much linoleic acid eating snack foods with safflower and sunflower oil. Avoiding trans fat is important (we'll discuss this in a moment), but replacing it with an excess of these two oils, which becomes DGLA, causes pain, sticky blood cells, weak vascular walls and is not the best option either. The critical point to the whole process, which is not widely known, is that the manmade, heated vegetable oil processing, called hydrogenation, creates trans fat, which also derails the process (more about this in Chapter 7). Not only does trans fat derail the process, but its bad effects last for a long time.

Trans Fat

Do you remember in science class when your teacher talked about the discovery of the half-life of uranium? Well, trans fat has a "half-life" too. Through research and experience, I have learned that the half-life of trans fat is 51 days. That may or may not seem like a long time, but you need to understand how it works. When you eat a bag of chips, a deep-fried donut, cream-filled cookies or anything with partially hydrogenated fat, it takes your body 51 days to properly metabolize and eliminate HALF of it. In another 51 days, HALF of that, 25 percent of the original amount, is still impacting body function. That's 102 days—over three months—and you still haven't processed all of the trans fat you just ate! If you are eating trans fat every day—and you are if you eat snack foods, prepackaged foods and deep-fried foods—imagine how much trans fat is congesting your body from years of this eating pattern. That's a pretty nauseating thought. Take two deep breaths and read this again.

Now you can call your old college roommate and tell him you know why little Joey has ADHD, or why you have depression and are not responding to medication, or why your auntie has Alzheimer's and is failing quickly—all of these conditions are precipitated by trans fat. Now do you see how big this really is?! Researchers—out of haste, ignorance and greed—have most people believing that margarine, which is made with trans fat, is better than butter. Do you remember the show of hands at my speaking event? No one, in all reality at this time, knows that what they are eating is silently and slowly killing them.

Let's continue; hang in there!

The Dairy Diet Myth

This next point will require you to be honest about how your body feels, and may just be a revelation for you. What I need to add to your understanding is that arachidonic acid, with its negative results, can be directly sourced, without processing, from dairy, red meat, mollusks and shell fish. These particular items can directly become arachidonic acid and processed to PG2. Clinically, I strongly encourage my patients to be conscious of dairy consumption and pain. Yes, you read right. The white-mustache dairy campaign promotes aches, pain and limited motion of the body. Dairy industry claims that drinking milk helps you lose weight have also proven false. *Obesity*, the official journal of The Obesity Society, captured this well:

> "Drink milk . . . Lose weight!" say the ads. The dairy industry has created an entire "Healthy Weight with Milk" campaign to boost sales. What's the evidence? Most of it came from a researcher who has a patent on the claim that dairy foods aid weight loss.
>
> In a new study—the largest so far—a high-dairy diet didn't help people lose weight. Twenty-three obese patients on 1,500-calorie diets who were randomly assigned to consume four servings of dairy a day lost no more weight or body fat after six months than 22 others who consumed one serving a day.
>
> What to do: Low-fat (or non-fat) milk, yogurt, and cheese can help lower blood pressure and boost calcium intake. But don't expect them to keep you slim.[1]

This direct sourcing of arachidonic acid, which makes PG2, the pain-causing prostaglandin, can be accelerated by trans fat consumption, insulin, alcohol, food coloring and preservatives (see Chart #2). The same process is inhibited by cortisone, bioflavonoids, turmeric in mustard, boswellia (an herb) and aspirin. Now you can see why what you eat has a direct impact on how you feel. The reason you are supposed to eat your five servings of fruits and vegetables a day is to promote pain relief and control PG2. Eating your basic fast-food meal depletes vitamins and minerals, sabotaging the heart-healthy and pain-relieving PG1, thus inviting pain into your body. I require all of my patients to keep a journal of what they eat so that they can see the correlation between what they are putting into their bodies and the pain they feel. I empower them with information so that they can be proactive contributors to a healthy lifestyle.

They quickly see that their results are directly affected by their choices. Some make the recommended changes and experience a higher quality of life, while others stay in denial and subsequently continue to suffer. It is always interesting after special holidays or on Mondays after big weekends of bad eating. My patients are experiencing pain, rationalizing the "small" piece of pie or "little" cookie as they indicate with hand gestures the small but lethal quantity of dietary "deviation" they imposed on their bodies.

Enough about that. It is time to move on to the other essential fat. We are not completely finished with linoleic acid, but I will bring it all together at the end of the next section.

Summary of Linoleic Acid

- It is essential for life and must be consumed.
- It is used to create and support bodily functions for optimal health.

- It requires calcium, magnesium, zinc, enzymes and quality-sourced whole-food B vitamins and B6 to evolve to PG1 or to arachidonic acid and PG2.

- It develops into pain-relieving, non-sticking blood cell PG1 or, if consumed too liberally, causes PG2 and pain and sticky blood cells.

- Its metabolic steps are detoured by sugar, alcohol, insulin, aspirin, food additives, minerals and enzymes.

- Its metabolic steps are sabotaged by trans fat intake.

- There is evidence-based experience from evaluations of diet journals that linoleic acid is more than adequately consumed in the current American daily diet pattern and, in many cases, almost too much of the "healthy" fat is consumed.

- It is sourced from most nuts and seeds, and from safflower and sunflower oils.

Summary of Non-Essential Arachidonic Acid

- It can be created from processing linoleic acid.

- It is directly sourced from the diet through dairy, meat, mollusk and shellfish consumption.

- It can evolve to PG2, which is pain creating and blood cell adhering.

- PG2 formation is inhibited by aspirin, COX inhibitors, bioflavonoids, vitamin C, cortisone, selected fat, turmeric and boswellia.

- PG2 formation is accelerated by trans fat, insulin, alcohol and food additives.

ALPHA-LINOLENIC ACID

Alpha-linolenic acid, or ALA, is the second essential fat, or fatty acid. The activity of ALA is comparable to its counterpart, linoleic acid, with a few exceptions. First, ALA is not normally consumed in the typical American diet. It requires a metabolic pathway that starts with items including flaxseeds, mixed greens, greens and walnuts, among other foods. Just as linoleic acid requires, these precursor foods need to go through steps with quality-sourced ingredients, including enzymes, calcium, magnesium, zinc, whole-food B vitamins and B6 (see Chart #3). The process can be inhibited by insulin, alcohol, food additives and deficiencies of vitamins, minerals and enzymes precipitated by anti-nutrients like sugar and stress. Trans fat sabotages the metabolic process, as it does for linoleic acid.

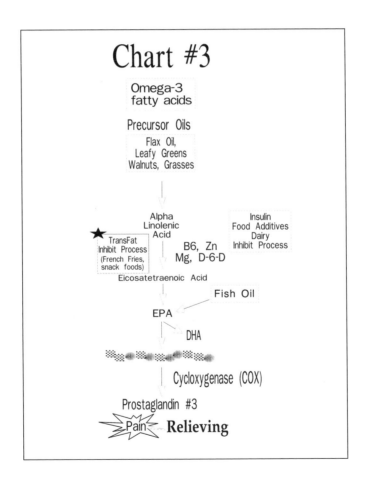

EPA and DHA

ALA continues on to become several very important long-chain fats that are needed for heart and brain/nerve health. The first is eicosapentaenoic acid, or EPA. EPA is the fat you will hear about being suggested as "heart smart." It can be directly sourced from marine (or "ocean fish") sources or from the pathway I just described, called the alpha-linolenic acid pathway, or ALA pathway for short. The other long-chain fat is called docosahexaenoic acid, or DHA. DHA is needed for proper brain and nervous system function. A research study I conducted with a group of participants overwhelmingly suggested that the breakdown of DHA through the ALA pathway, precipitated by trans fat consumption, was the primary cause of ADHD, ADD and hyperactivity. (See *Dr. Bob's Guide to Stop ADHD in 18 days*, Chapter 18.) ALA progresses on to become another prostaglandin, or fat tissue hormone, named prostaglandin 3, or PG3, which, like PG1, is a pain-relieving, non-sticking blood cell prostaglandin.

Controversy over fat metabolism is common. As I've said, the observations I share here with you were gathered from real people with actual life issues and not from experimental lab animals or controlled human research environments. As also mentioned, taking COX inhibitors, aspirin and the like does not correct the problem but only hides the symptoms. Pain must be managed through lifestyle changes, specifically through eating foods that enhance health.

Aspirin is consumed by the tens of millions each year in the United States. But that doesn't make it good for you! Hormone replacement therapy was also taken by the millions—and people died. COX inhibitors for pain relief (see Chapter 5) destroyed thousands of people's lives in their short but profitable existence. Millions of dollars were spent by direct marketing to promote the use of Vioxx® before it was ultimately withdrawn over safety concerns. Doctors and patients appeared to have the mindset that new is better. Similar consequences of poor health are occurring right now, and will continue until someone takes a position and informs the public that, with many drugs on the market, *you are tricking your body.*

Aspirin works by inhibiting the formation of PG2, the pain-causing prostaglandin, resulting in pain relief, yes, but *not in healing.* Aspirin also interferes with the formation of PG1 and PG3, which act much like aspirin by causing blood cells to repel or not stick together; they are also pain relieving. So, what the research scientist in the pharmaceutical industry doesn't want you to know is that taking aspirin, physiologically, is just a temporary patch for a deeper problem. The aspirin makers generate billions of dollars and are aware that aspirin is media driven and not the answer for everyone. That is why we have the COX inhibitors and other pain-relieving options for the estimated 86 million Americans who live in chronic pain. Aspirin does not promote natural function in the human body. It is wrong! And aspirin's side effects may be causing some of your subpar bodily functions, though you or your physician may have not yet made the connection. As I mentioned earlier in the book, aspirin slows bone fracture healing and could be a factor in osteoporosis. Now, that doesn't mean to throw out all of your aspirin. I am not recommending that you stop aspirin without investigating your current health status, which is why I suggest to our patients and clients worldwide that they have their EFA levels tested, including their arachidonic acid levels (pain and "sticky cell" producers). So, then, what is my message here? Be aware.

Pain relief–driven treatment programs create massive revenues in our medically minded economy. The patients who seek natural drugless care are capable of achieving a pain-free lifestyle without the side effects of prescription or over-the-counter medication. But to live drug free without pain, you will need to modify your diet to achieve optimal health—by removing refined sugar and trans fat from your diet and by limiting dairy, red meat and alcohol. Can you do it? Yes, you can! Knowledge is power.

Healthy Fat

In my practice, I have seen and treated the devastation of kidney and liver disease caused by pain medication prescribed by a physician with the instructions to take it "like candy." I have seen organ transplants as a result of pain medication stressing the system. Cortisone, prednisone and other steroids can, over time, be disfiguring. I recommend to my patients organic-sourced, high lignan omega processed flax oil or gel capsules and I see consistent, long-term results.

The public is encouraged to consume marine life for sources of EPA and DHA. My patient diet journals suggest that as a group we consume similar levels of marine products today as we did in the 1970s. Therefore, I do not believe more deep-water fish is the one-shot, easy to "pop a natural pill" answer to heart health challenges. The reason you will read about salmon and salmon capsules and other marine foods as sources of EPA and DHA for the heart and brain is because nearly all researchers believe the body is not genetically capable of making enough of these long-chain fats. But taking salmon capsules as a consistent fat supplement may, in fact, thin your blood too much, potentially resulting in a stroke or internal bleeding. If you are taking these supplements regularly, I suggest having your EFAs tested to assess what specific oils you would do best to focus on. And I would not—under any circumstances—take flax or any marine-sourced oil capsules, including salmon capsules, while you are taking blood thinners without being monitored by your health care provider.

Here is a question for you. Why did we have a human body that worked well 30, 40 or 50 years ago and yet is now not making enough EPA and DHA? The answer is two-fold. First, trans fat sabotages your body's ability to make EPA and DHA from, as discussed, 51 days and continuing for 102 days. Second, the source of minerals, vitamins and enzymes in our environment is so pitifully low that Americans are mineral and vitamin deficient. Vitamins, minerals and enzymes are also needed to have success in the ALA process. "But I take my One-a-Day A-to-Z tablet packed with everything I need!" you exclaim. That may be, but what I know and what other natural practitioners know is that these vitamins are usually synthetic. They are processed, isolated and fractionalized. They are chemical compounds created in a lab and do not always fit into the cell structure of the body. I can tell you this with confidence because I see real people every day who bring me their boxes, bags and plastic containers of mega ballistic vitamins and still feel lousy. Generally, low-dosage, cold-processed, food-sourced products are best. If you take supplements and you're not progressing, you may want to contemplate making some modifications. In my practice, I use whole-food-based supplements that have not been isolated or fractionalized to large or small sizes.

Even with all of the technology available today, there are particles not yet discovered in whole foods that are required for life. We have an ever increasing amount of epidemic sicknesses in our developed Western cultures because we have over-processed our foods, including vitamins and mineral supplements, making them less effective. Natural function is based on low-dose levels of nutrients similar to the composition found in food; cell function is very specific in following the patterns set by nature. For example, an orange naturally has about 25 mg of vitamin C. We are bombarded by well-meaning physicians and magazine articles telling us to take 500 mg of vitamin C in the form of ascorbic acid (which is not the natural complex form of vitamin C but the fractionalized version) to fight and fend off the "cold and flu" viruses; that would be the equivalent of 20 oranges! Does that sound like something you would want to do?

You would have to take a pill the size of a Ping-Pong ball to get the full benefit of a complex natural 500 mg vitamin C tablet using that mindset of a proper dosage. We can actually get too many milligrams and units of "synthetic" vitamins that can confuse the body. Therefore, bigger is not always better when it comes to the constituents in your vitamins. The ALA pathway requires the right ingredients, in the right amounts, to function. Nature has done this for us. As Hippocrates said, "Let food be your medicine and medicine be your food."

One consolation here is that synthetic vitamins, especially the larger ones, make awesome slingshot ammunition! They leave a mark when you hit the target. Go on, try it. Have some fun!

Summary of Alpha-Linolenic Acid

- ALA is one of the essential fats you must consume.
- It is sourced indirectly from flax, mixed greens, green foods and selected nuts and seeds.
- It evolves to EPA for heart health and DHA for brain and nervous system function.
- It is processed to become prostaglandin 3, which is pain relieving and non–blood cell sticking.
- It requires calcium, magnesium, zinc, B vitamins, B6 and enzymes to process.
- It is inhibited by insulin, food additives, alcohol, aspirin, COX inhibitors and deficiencies in enzymes, vitamins and minerals.
- ALA is sabotaged by trans fat.
- Analysis of patient diet journals indicates that ALA is lacking from the standard American diet.

FACTS ABOUT FAT - ACTION STEPS

☐ Avoid foods that have trans fat or partially hydrogenated oils in the ingredients.

☐ Focus on consuming a variety of cold-processed oils. Flax and olive oil are two to have on your list, but limit safflower and sunflower oils.

☐ Dairy, red meat, mollusks and shell fish should be limited, as they create pain.

☐ Take up to one tablespoon of flax oil per 100 pounds of body weight. Do not take flax and marine oil without having your EFAs evaluated with a blood spot test.

☐ Take a whole-food multiple vitamin and mineral supplement.

☐ Use rice, egg white or pumpkin powder protein instead of whey-based products.

☐ Marine-based oils are best from small fish like anchovies or sardines; avoid tuna and large fish oils.

NOTES

5

NO MORE PAIN

It is estimated that 50 to 80 million people in our population suffer with pain on a daily basis, creating a multibillion-dollar pharmaceutical industry. There are many reasons for pain. As you've been learning in this book (and which few Americans know), what you eat will have an impact on pain levels in your body. As we've discussed, the consumption of trans fat is one of several factors that promotes pain: 1) by increasing the production of the fat tissue hormone prostaglandin 2 (PG2) and/or 2) by inhibiting the body's ability to make pain-relieving prostaglandin 1 (PG1) and prostaglandin 3 (PG3).

Pain is an integral part of normal bodily function. When a body part is damaged by injury from a fall, motor vehicle accident, sports injury, etc., chemicals are released to stimulate the healing process. Your body is specifically designed to repair itself. We are a self-healing organism and pain is part of the repair process. Pain can also occur because of postural breakdown during the aging process. Aging tissues are compressed, stretched, squeezed and moved, creating a bombardment to the supporting structures. This results in a chemical release response, causing repair from an injury to be slower and more painful.

CHRONIC PAIN

Chronic pain syndromes are a common unresolved dilemma. The million-dollar question for chronic pain sufferers is: What is causing the pain? This is the most obvious question to answer, but is, from my point of view, the one that has not yet been addressed—largely due to the ignorance of the general public and the greed of those in the conventional pain relief market. The accepted mindset is that it is easier to take a pill to relieve pain than it is to make lifestyle changes to alleviate the pain at its root cause.

Pain is real. I have seen thousands of patients who have been in pain for years find relief in a short time period without adding a new medication. Pain at the cellular level, as I mentioned in Chapter 4, is caused by uncontrolled chemical responses precipitated by eating foods that inhibit PG1 and/or PG3 production so they cannot be a part of the pain-relieving equation. Another factor in the pain-relieving equation is eating *too much* of the foods that create PG1 (safflower and sunflower oils, snack and convenience foods). When these are in overabundance in the body, PG2 is created, adding pain instead of relieving it (see Chart #2 on page 53). This information is not currently commonly known or understood, or perhaps, because it seems so simple, it is just ignored. After all, many still think margarine is good!

WHAT FOODS CAUSE PAIN?

What foods cause pain? Foods that stop PG1 and PG3. The number one and two foods are trans fat and sugar, which are in nearly all prepackaged snack food products. Trans fat, remember, prolongs pain because of its 51-day "half-life." Your body is concentrating on trying to metabolize the trans fat that inhibits the pain-relieving prostaglandins and goes out of balance. You need to consume a 1:1 ratio of omega-6 fats, which produce PG1, and omega-3 fats,

which produce PG3. A ratio of 4:1 is a practical goal to begin relieving some of the pain. The "four" part of the ratio is the amount
of pain-producing oils, which most people consume in their diet
via convenience or fast food items. The "one" is the ration of food
choices that metabolize to the pain-relieving PG3. Though not the
ideal ratio, with a 4:1 consumption of pain-causing to pain-relieving
foods, you at least won't have the same potentially relentless pain
ruling your life.

Prostaglandin #1 Primarily sourced from Omega 6 Fats	Prostaglandin #2 Primarily sourced from Omega 6 Fats and directly from the following:	Prostaglandin #3 Primarily sourced from Omega 3 Fats
Primrose Oil Black currant Oil Borage Oil Safflower Oil Sunflower Oil	Dairy Red Meat Mollusks Shellfish	Flax Oil Greens Algae Selected nuts Marine–directly sourced from fish

When the ratio is anywhere from 1:1 to 4:1, there is a fairly even
distribution of pain-relieving and pain-causing chemicals. But a
much more common occurrence in America with our addiction to
snack foods, where the average annual consumption is well over 30
pounds per person, the ratio is more like 20:1. Yes, the public eats
20 times the amount of foods that cause pain versus relieve pain.
*I also want to gently remind you here that the "good" oils like safflower
and sunflower oils, which metabolize to pain-relieving PG1, when eaten
in abundance translate to PG2* (see Charts #1 and #2). *This is a built-in
"safety valve" to protect you from bleeding to death.* With these statistics,
it's no wonder the pain-relief industry is so enormous! That huge
disparity also contributes to blood vessel inflammation with high
LDL cholesterol as well as other behavioral, emotional and memory
problems (see *Dr. Bob's Guide to Stop ADHD in 18 Days*).

Take a look at snack food and energy bar labels. You can easily see why what we are eating is causing our pain. Most of our snack foods contain dairy, sugar and trans fat, and many of us overeat meat, which adds to the pain. Excessive PG2 can create an environment increasing not only pain and vascular disease, but also cancer, decay, immune system dysfunctions, free radicals (think oxidation damage, like rusting) and Alzheimer's (see Chart #4). Pain relievers work by interfering with the production of PG2. But when the PG2 pathway is altered artificially by adding your daily aspirin and/or other pain relievers, you are altering normal physiology. There is a cascade effect that also changes the ratio of PG1 and PG3, resulting in a temporary increase in the pain-relieving factors and a ratio favoring PG3. The main problem with this is that the constant altering of fat metabolism has a negative impact on your detoxifying organs, the kidneys and liver.

Taking medication to stop pain without thinking about what is causing the pain is similar to taking pharmaceuticals to lower LDL cholesterol without attempting to correct the cause. A side note: The pharmaceutical companies, to be fair, do actually encourage positive dietary changes in some of their advertising and marketing campaigns. And the public is aware of the need to avoid cholesterol foods like cheese, ice cream and red meat, which is a step in the right direction. The real cause of high cholesterol and pain, however, is sugar, vitamin and mineral deficiencies and trans fat, and these issues are not being presented.

Now, you know that trans fat can precipitate pain and that eating too many trans fat alternatives like safflower and sunflower oils can also cause pain because they are part of the omega-6 family. Ratio, remember, is the key. Omega-6 fats are not bad for you, but the amount must be balanced with omega-3 fats for our bodies to function properly. Margarine is almost purely an omega-6 fatty acid and

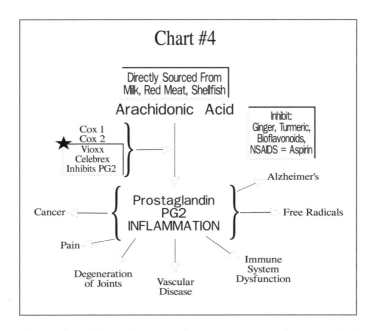

Chart #4

Directly Sourced From
Milk, Red Meat, Shellfish

Arachidonic Acid

Inhibit:
Ginger, Turmeric,
Bioflavonoids,
NSAIDS = Aspirin

Cox 1
Cox 2
Vioxx
Celebrex
Inhibits PG2

Prostaglandin
PG2
INFLAMMATION

Cancer

Pain

Degeneration
of Joints

Vascular
Disease

Alzheimer's

Free Radicals

Immune
System
Dysfunction

a trans fat. It should not be anywhere near your diet—including in the snack and convenience foods you pick up at the counter, at the service station and at the ball game vendors. Peanuts . . . Popcorn . . . Pain!

WHAT YOU CAN DO

You have now been empowered to know what causes pain. So what do you do? First, you avoid pain-promoting sugar, dairy, trans fats and even sweet fruits like bananas, raisins, grapes, pineapple and dried fruits. I have discovered over time that patients who eat fruits focus on the sweet ones. A pain-free choice would include pears, plums and apples. Next, introduce omega-3 foods like mixed green salads, green beans, walnuts, flax oil, flaxseeds and flax powder into your diet. Also consume vitamin B–rich foods and minerals, including zinc, magnesium and calcium. Alfalfa is a good source of all of these minerals. Work on replacing dairy with rice and almond beverage products. In my practice, I do not encourage soy products, particularly not for men. Soy can deplete zinc and encourage aluminum to remain in the body, neither of which promotes optimal health. Choose to eat a variety of fresh, raw organic vegetables and the pain-free fruits mentioned above. Grains have a ratio of 20:1 or greater of omega-6 to omega-3 oils, and grain-fed animals have ratios above 4:1. In the pain equation, these should be referred to as pro-inflammatory foods. Therefore, please notice food packaging labels that say "grass fed," as these items tend to have more pain-free content than the grain-, pen- and barn-fed sources. Becoming well informed and label savvy is crucial to your long-term health journey.

If you are taking a COX inhibiting drug, how does this affect you? COX is an acronym for cyclooxygenase. Much has been discussed about COX-1 and COX-2, the two different COX enzymes. It has also been proposed that there is a third COX enzyme, COX-3. The difference between the first two is straightforward. COX-1 is involved in bodily functions like stomach protection and kidney function. In contrast, COX-2 is not involved at all in tissue function or balance; instead, it is induced or active after tissue injury.

There is confusion revolving around COX-2 being an inflammatory enzyme. It is not. COX-2 is an enzyme that is induced by tissue injury. The response is dependent on the nature of the fatty acids present in the cell membranes. This is huge, huge, HUGE. The response is determined by what you are eating! If COX-2 acts with arachidonic acid, the outcome will be the synthesis of PG2, which produces pain, reduces blood flow and causes blood platelets to stick. If the fat to make PG1 or DGLA is present, there is a non-inflammatory response. If the fat to make PG3 or EPA is present, there is a non-inflammatory response. Pharmacology articles and pathology texts do not make this distinction, which is why the public is led to believe that COX-2 enzymes are inherently inflammatory.[1] The bad effects of the COX inhibiting medication is a travesty. I have personally witnessed and talked with patients who have had spinal cord strokes directly related to this type of pain reliever. Tens of thousands of people have been harmed.

We literally eat ourselves into a state of inflammation and pain and then have to take medications as a counteractive measure. The excessive inflammation created by the overabundance of omega-6 fatty acids is also thought to be the main reason for the development of cancer, heart disease, stroke and other inflammatory conditions. The headlines in major newspapers consistently report the new information being released on the dangers of COX medications, plus aspirin and other non-steroidal anti-inflammatory drugs. A word of caution: Think twice before you put a pain reliever in your body.

NO MORE PAIN – ACTIONS STEPS

☐ Eat a variety of fats and oils that are cold pressed. Consume limited amounts of snack and convenience foods with safflower and sunflower oil. Concentrate on using olive and flax oils. Do not heat flax.

☐ Use rice and almond beverages as an alternative to dairy-related products and beverages. Look at labels; sugar in any product creates pain.

☐ Focus on pears, plums and apples for pain relief.

☐ Trans fat is also called partially hydrogenated oil. Look at the front label; if it has "0 Grams Trans Fat" don't assume it's true. Look at the ingredients and make sure there is no hydrogenated oil.

☐ If you have pain, add one tablespoon of flax oil per 100 pounds of body weight to your supplement regime.

☐ Do not mix aspirin and flax or any fish or marine sourced oils—
    salmon, tuna, cod, calamari, anchovy or sardine, as all of these
    thin your blood.

☐ If you notice bruising on your arms or hands, evaluate how many
    blood-thinning foods and medications you are taking. Talk to
    your prescribing physician or pharmacist.

NOTES _____

_____

_____

_____

_____

_____

_____

_____

_____

_____

_____

_____

_____

_____

_____

_____

_____

_____

_____

_____

_____

6

REACH AND MAINTAIN YOUR NORMAL WEIGHT

Achieving an optimal weight level given the fast-paced life-style most of us have today appears to be eternally elusive. There always seems to be another book or magazine article suggesting that if you eat one food and/or avoid another, your pounds will magically slip away never to return. How many times have you been down that road?

Over my career, I have seen countless people in this boat, gaining then losing hundreds of pounds, only to gain them again. One thing I know for sure, losing weight and keeping it off for good does not have to get harder as you get chronologically older. I have helped innumerable patients lose weight and keep it off. The critical key is to allow the body to *heal itself* then watch the pounds naturally melt away. There is no magic bullet, just a few natural health care protocols that must be followed:

1. Build a foundation on a solidly functioning hormonal or endocrine system
2. Detoxify the cleansing organs
3. Avoid toxic substances

I have had many patients tell me that they really watch what they eat, and have been disciplined, but the weight just stays. Is that you? If so, what is going on? A consistently obese body that does not respond long term to selected food avoidance and portion control is, generally, an unhealthy system. The body, as a defense mechanism to protect you, will not permit the uncontrolled release of fat because it is either being saved for a future time or the content in the fat or adipose tissue is so toxic that releasing it results in a damaging response. You see, abdominal or visceral fat not only produces estrogen, but it is also a common depot for synthetic estrogens and other environmental toxins. We'll talk about estrogen in just a moment.

Your body protects you by storing toxins in your fat; the fat cells act as a literal "hazardous dumping site." In fact, that's what cellulite really is—a storehouse of fat toxins. Once you have the toxic fats in your body, and if you continue living a lifestyle where you constantly accumulate more toxins from processed foods, beverages, body lotions, creams and even medications, your body has no other choice but to continue the storage process in the deep recesses of your thighs, buttocks and abdomen. You are literally burying what appears like those 55-gallon drums with the skull and crossbones, usually reserved for isolation in some remote location, only now they are being stored in YOU.

This reality often strikes when it could already be too late, and you are told you have cancer! Toxic buildup, as you'll read in Chapter 15 on the thyroid, can also sabotage normal hormonal function, causing subpar thyroid function and liver compromise with stasis issues. As a man, you could experience prostate swelling, headaches, coughing and sinus congestion with post-nasal drip; these are signals that your body is reacting to toxic buildup.

BODY FAT DISTRIBUTION

I am a student of "body watching" and have seen clearly that people come in all shapes and sizes. Interestingly, there are visible patterns of fat distribution on the bodies of people who have various organs that are toxic, overloaded and burned out. Following are the most common body types for both genders, with men tending to have the "toxic liver" body type most often.

The Thyroid Type

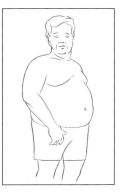

Some people carry their weight all over the body, which suggests thyroid gland distress. These same individuals may have cold hands and feet, high cholesterol and be constipated in addition to some of the other body signals discussed in Chapter 15 on the thyroid. They may have small cherry-like nodules on their skin, cherry hemangiomas, suggesting estrogen saturation. Common factors that can create this scenario include:

- modern chemicals designed to enhance the production of the food chain and household conveniences that also impair and affect the recipient (i.e., you, the consumer)

- xenohormones, found in cleaning products, aerosols, lotions, fabrics, paints and many common domestic items. These are part of a toxic chain that interferes with normal hormone function.

- elevated estrogen levels. Whether they are natural or sourced from chemicals, high estrogen levels impair thyroid function and congest the liver/gallbladder relationship, resulting in stagnant gallbladder bile flow and congestion.

When the thyroid is hampered in doing its work, you will see an overall-body weight gain. That is why consuming conventionally sourced animal products, usually containing synthetic estrogen to "fatten" the animal tissue, has created an enormous challenge for unsuspecting consumers. Clean machines (i.e., our bodies) always work better with the least amount of outside chemicals.

Chlorine and fluorine added to the municipal water supply in our communities are a part of the water supply in your house, apartment or other living space. These two less-than-health-promoting compounds are everywhere. You will find them in your kitchen sink, bathrooms and shower stall. Any time you open the tap to get water from your sink and then use it to wash or prepare meals, you are consuming potentially toxic compounds. The government, by the way, recently lowered legal levels of fluorine in tap water because there is so much of it now that people are getting discoloring or mottling of their teeth. Bromine, another toxic substance found in pools and hot tubs, also creates an extra lethal burden for the body and the liver/gallbladder detoxification system. This trio of chemical compounds competes with iodine for receptors. Iodine is used by every cell in the body, including the thyroid, which is critically important for optimal weight. Aggravating the situation is that iodine deficiencies are very common in our general dietary food patterns. In fact, 72 percent of the world's population has insufficient iodine. The result is a full figure or thyroid body type.

The Adrenal Type

Stress, as discussed in earlier chapters, whether caused by emotional or physical means, affects the adrenal glands. You'll recall that the adrenal glands supply many critical hormones for our existence, one of which is cortisol (cortisone). When you are under stress, your cortisol levels are up and you will have a tendency for the carbohydrates you eat (cookies, pasta, grain snacks, donuts, etc.) to be converted to body fat. What is significant is that "naked sweets" (items that are strictly carbohydrates or refined grain products with "sugar added" and no protein to slow the burn or consumption process down) will result in cortisol being released as a negative feedback loop to stop the rampage of insulin that is simultaneously being secreted by the pancreas. Patients who are stressed and eating a lot of carbohydrates and stimulants 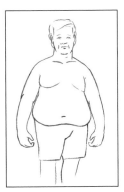 tend to have more of their extra tissue hanging around as a "spare tire" around the waist—the adrenal pattern.

The Liver or Big Belly Type

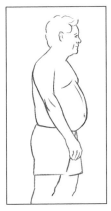 Intentional or unaware consumption of toxic food and drink, including artificial sweeteners, taste enhancers, preservatives and even prescription medications, can overload the very important liver-detoxification system. Your liver has many job descriptions. A key function of the liver is to dispose of unwanted and unnecessary substances. Someone who has a huge protruding belly with "humpty-dumpty" bean-pole legs will generally have a liver that has expanded and is in a compromised state and currently not working to its full potential. Here, there is fat and fluid hanging over the belt. This particular body type will require real discipline because addictive choices have created this downwardly spiraling state of health.

The Estrogen-Saturation Type

One body shape that I am starting to see more of in males of all ages is literally the "female body type" that can develop at any age once the secondary male sexual characteristics appear. This type can be

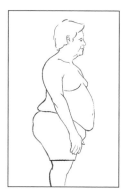 considered an estrogen-saturation body type. When a young boy, adolescent or adult male are exposed to excessive amounts of estrogen—and we are living in a "sea of estrogen" now, where the hormone can be found in unfiltered tap water, canned foods, soy products, conventional meat products and chemicals from lawn and plant herbicide applications—their body responds with female characteristics, commonly observed in males as an increase in the size of breast tissue. All you have to do is to look around at the pool or exercise clubs. I have observed that men today over 55 often have more estrogen in their system than their female mates of the same age do. This is a real travesty, the extent of which very few realize.

The real challenge with fat distribution is that you can have a combination of body types due to hormonal mis-cues along with the over-consumption of sweets, lack of exercise and toxic reservoirs. Adding to this scenario is that fat cells can create estrogen. Now this is a double-edged sword for the general population, because today we are dealing with fake estrogens or xenohormones in unprecedented amounts and these mimic estrogen. Estrogen dominance creates havoc in the body and stresses the liver/gallbladder. You need the liver to process the hormones in the body. The alteration of this loop escalates the fat-accumulation dilemma. Since society as a whole is being exposed to more estrogen than we need or can handle, this is a huge potential epidemic that literally feeds and expands the obesity men and boys need to contend with.

RESTARTING THE HORMONE LOOP TO BEGIN LOSING WEIGHT

An exhausted system, with hormonal depletion, congested toxification of organs and a general overall poor state of health will not reduce excess fat until the body is healthy. If you are struggling and dealing with excessive fat, you need to become healthy and not start another fad diet; otherwise, you will be chasing a state that is not attainable. Now, you cannot get impatient and you do not want to get caught up with the "in moderation" style of eating. No cookies means NO cookies, not even small ones. I don't care how "healthy" they are. The carbohydrates in them will throw a wrench into your system and thus your progress.

The answer to your problem starts with normalizing the hormonal system in your body. If you do not restart that loop, you will not achieve your optimal health; therefore, you will not lose weight permanently. The hypothalamus, your body's CEO, tells the rest of the body what to do. I have seen from experience that it can take anywhere from six months to a year to refuel and restart this hormone loop. If you have had your gallbladder removed, it will take longer because the liver has been compromised, and the liver is the hormone recycle depot.

To begin rebuilding their hormonal foundation, I start male patients with the food-supplement pillar, recommending several items to support and restructure the overall hormone system (pituitary, thyroid, adrenal and testes):

- I recommend products called "glandulars" that sustain brain health by supporting the pituitary and hypothalamus loop. The general protocol is three to six of each supplement— some for the brain and others for endocrine support. The glandulars I use have been developed and restricted by adhering and being compliant to FDA guidelines. They are available only through licensed health care providers. Because you do not want to start taking an item that does not promote health or fails to get to the real root of the problem, talk to your natural doctor to get a product from a quality source. There are a variety of companies that create very good products that support hormonal health using the technology of glandular cell therapy. I have taken glandulars myself in the past, and currently take a product for the thyroid, adrenal and testes.

■ I have also found that most people who need to lose weight need a full spectrum of oil. That would encompass the omega-3, -6 and -9 fats, the fats that are, in part (the -3 and -6), used to create PG1 and PG2. That's why I like black currant seed oil; it is a complete oil that has all of the basics to support your hormonal health. I would encourage you to look for a brand that is labeled "mixed EFAs"—meaning mixed essential fatty acids. Choose organic items, as they eliminate the extra burden to the body of the chemicals that are often used to extract oils from their sources. Hexane, for example, is commonly used to extract soy oil from the beans. Pressed oils, on the other hand, are just that—they are squeezed. Use the oil for a minimum of three months to jump-start your system. I use some type of oil every day, either on my salad or "down the hatch" with my other morning supplements.

■ I also suggest that you follow the Page Diet plan, found in Chapter 17, as a template of what to eat and what not to. Put your focus on eating cruciferous vegetables: broccoli, cabbage, cauliflower, Brussels sprouts and kale; these foods tend to counter the negative impact from the synthetic estrogens you are constantly being exposed to. They are best consumed either raw, steamed or sautéed in olive or coconut oil. If you are focusing on these food items, add a whole-food iodine product starting with a minimum of 3 mg a day, as they tend to antagonize iodine. I personally take 12 mg of iodine daily. You will learn more about iodine in other sections of the book.

How do you know when you have a proper hormone balance? Well, an objective approach would be to have a tissue-hair mineral analysis and look at the selenium level, which tends to be low with a stressed pituitary. Another marker would be to check your TSH, T3 and T4, revealing thyroid function, before you start the process. A low TSH is also often associated with a stressed pituitary. In my practice, I add a whole-food vitamin E, at a minimum of three low-dosage tablets daily, to increase the selenium levels. Also, if you start to see the browning of your skin, or are getting brown spots, this is a signal that your pituitary and liver do not have enough vitamin E. The liver has everything to do with skin lesions. Do not use synthetic vitamin E.

IDENTIFYING YOUR BODY TYPE

Before you take the complete "body type" quiz towards the end of this chapter, there are several questions you can ask up front that will quickly tell you if your liver and gallbladder are drawn into your weight challenge. If these organs are congested or compromised, you will discover that that could be the cause of your slow weight loss progress (common body signals of gallbladder/liver involvement include digestive distress with green peppers, onions, cucumbers and/or radishes). If the answers to these preliminary questions are yes, you might want to read Chapter 8 on the liver and then focus your attention on cleansing the whole body by eating according to the Page Diet (see Chapter 17).

So, as a pre-test, go through the questions below. If you check ANY of the seven points listed here, you do not need to go through the Body Type Quiz—you already have your answer: You need foods that support the liver! You would do best eating at least one-half of a red apple daily to support bile flow through your liver, one-third cup of organic beets (grated fresh or baked) and one medium carrot to support liver function. These three items comprise "Dr. Bob's ABCs."

Additionally, if you've had your gallbladder removed, taking a bile salt–based whole-food product should be a part of your daily protocol. At 500,000 per year in the United States alone, gallbladder removal is quite common! That's the equivalent of five "football bowl" stadiums. Wrap your brain around that! When a patient has had gallbladder surgery, it's a red flag to me that this person has compromised liver function, poor digestion and a slow-burning, fat-gaining metabolism.

☐ Have you had your gallbladder removed?

☐ History of gallstones?

☐ Can't lose weight on high-protein diets (e.g., Atkins)?

☐ Dislike consuming lots of heavy protein-type foods?

☐ Inability to digest fatty or greasy foods, especially at night?

☐ History of liver problems?

☐ Protruding, distended belly (i.e., potbelly)?

☐ Right shoulder blade region pain?

In this case, eating pastries and donuts only torpedoes the ability to get well. **Trans fat, when studied and monitored, has statistically been shown to increase your weight over time.** Research on test animals reveals that trans fat–fed animals had an up to 7 percent increase in weight compared to animals that were fed olive oil instead of the trans fat.[1] This could be correlated to the findings that the low-fat (trans fat) diet commonly consumed in America, which we were led to believe is healthy and a way to lose weight, is actually incorrect!

By following the protocols you have learned throughout this book, your overall system will be working in harmony. Your challenge, as being in command of your body's multitude of activities, is to control the desire for those items that create cravings for the sugar that releases insulin, which then crescendos into cortisol release, which then promotes fat deposits and the cannibalizing of muscle tissue for fuel, slowing weight loss. Three of the most significant insights, by far, that I can leave with you are: **1) Do not eat sugar, 2) avoid foods that have chemicals added and 3) avoid trans fat or partially hydrogenated oils.** Your body has to process each of these and looks at the man-tampered ones as foreign invaders. And the bottom line is that if you eat synthetic ingredients, you will have more challenges managing your weight; the liver will be compromised and, as you just read, you need an optimal functioning liver in your corner if you want to get rid of that belly.

I see so many people today who are extremely overweight, to the point that they can hardly walk, and I don't want you to become one or remain as one. If you want to be successful, your focus is to:

- ☐ Eat less, eat right. "Right" means eating protein and non-starchy veggies.

- ☐ Avoid trans fat, which in itself causes extra weight.

- ☐ Drink adequate pure water—at least a quart a day. Do not drink water with meals.

- ☐ Avoid all grains, and say no to alcohol (including wine).

- ☐ Maintain sufficient exercise and sleep patterns.

- ☐ Avoid stress and over-commitments.

As mentioned in an earlier chapter, in my practice I use a tool called the acoustic cardiogram. It transposes sound energy, made by the heart valves closing, into a mechanical graph. There are various patterns that can be observed. If we see minimal graph sounds, it indicates that there is a stressed hormonal system.

For patients who get this result, I prescribe a one-month detoxification program focusing on limited foods, with a colon cleanse and green food. Green food is a necessary factor promoting whole-body purification. So, the plan for the month would include protein, green food and a colon cleanser.

Upon completing the one-month cleanse and having your hormones pointed in the right direction, I assess the major hormonal organ needs. Often there is a combination of one or more. See Chapters 13 and 15 on adrenal and thyroid health. You need to follow the protocols in those chapters.

An important step is to rate the function of the hypothalamus and pituitary. These are not areas in the body that are generally monitored. As mentioned, a periodic hair analysis to monitor the selenium levels and the serum TSH in the thyroid profile is a subtle way to stay on track. Support your system with what you have learned. You may need to stay on the brain and hormonal glandular products I discussed at the beginning of the chapter because you may not be able to change your lifestyle and will need to continue to support all of your endocrine organs. The supplements I use with my patients have never caused any signals of toxic accumulation, and I have successfully used them since the early 1970s as both a patient and as a natural health doctor.

BODY TYPE QUIZ

DIRECTIONS: For each question below, circle the answer that best fits you. If you experience more than one symptom, circle the one that is most prominent.

1. Do you:
A. crave sweets, breads and pasta?
B. crave salt (pretzels, cheese puffs or salty peanuts) or chocolate?
C. crave deep-fried foods or potato chips?
D. crave ice cream, cream cheese, sour cream or milk?

2. Are you:
   A. often depressed or feeling hopeless?
   B. a worrier or often anxious and nervous?
   C. irritable, moody or grouchy in the morning?
   D. moody or irritable?

3. Do you:
   A. feel better on fruits and berries?
   B. need coffee or stimulants to wake up?
   C. experience a tight feeling over your right, lower stomach area or rib cage?
   D. experience constipation?

4. Do you have:
   A. brittle nails with vertical ridges?
   B. to wear sunglasses on a cloudy day?
   C. pain/tightness in right shoulder area?
   D. pain in right or left lower back/hip area?

5. Do you have:
   A. a weight problem more evenly distributed?
   B. a pendulous abdomen, meaning hanging, sagging and loose?
   C. a protruding abdomen (potbelly)?
   D. excess fat on thighs and hips and a lower stomach bulge?

6. Do you have:
   A. dry skin, especially hands and around elbows?
   B. swollen ankles; socks leave creases on ankles?
   C. flaky skin or dandruff in eyebrows and scalp?
   D. hair loss?

7. Do you have:
   A. indentations on both sides of your tongue where the tongue meets the teeth?
   B. atrophy (shrinkage) of the thigh muscles with difficulty getting up from a seated position?
   C. dark yellow urine?
   D. trouble sleeping through the night?

8. Do you have:
    A. a loss of hair on the outer third of the eyebrows?
    B. dizziness when getting up too quickly?
    C. hot or swollen feet?
    D. brain fog?

9. Do you have:
    A. to sleep with socks on at night because of feeling cold?
    B. chronic inflammation in body?
    C. headaches or head feels heavy in the morning?
    D. breasts that are getting larger or growing (i.e., "man boobs")

10. Do you have:
    A. puffiness around your eyes?
    B. an unusual feeling of being "out of breath" while climbing stairs?
    C. skin problems (psoriasis, eczema, brown spots)?
    D. low sex drive?

11. Do you have/Are you:
    A. excessive skin sagging under arms?
    B. twitching under or on top of left eyelid?
    C. not a morning person, yet feel more awake at night?
    D. cyclic weight gain

12. Do you:
    A. have dry hair and hair loss?
    B. wake up in the middle of the night (2 a.m. - 3 a.m.)?
    C. have a deep crevice (deep crease appearance) down the center of your tongue and/or a white film on your tongue?
    D. have an upper body that is thinner than your lower body?

13. Do you experience:
    A. a loss of the curly locks you had as a kid?
    B. cramps in the calves at night?
    C. more itching at night?
    D. water retention, "boggy" wrist, feeling swollen

14. Do you:
A. become excessively tired in the early evening (7:30 p.m. – 8 p.m.) and more awake in the early morning?
B. have a more active bladder at night than during the day?
C. have a yellow tint in the whites of your eyes?
D. consume nonorganic meat?

15. Do you have:
A. a lack of get-up-and-go (vitality)?
B. calcium issues or deposits—bursitis, tendonitis, kidney stones, heal spurs, early cataracts?
C. major moodiness if you skip a meal?
D. difficulty losing weight?

16. Do you have:
A. a history of being on low-calorie diets?
B. low tolerance for stressful situations, getting easily irritable and on edge?
C. stiffness and pain more in the right shoulder and right side of your neck?
D. pain and tightness inside the heels?

Count up the total of each:

Total A. Thyroid _____   **Total B. Adrenal** _____

Total C. Liver _____   **Total D. Hormone Imbalance** _____

Tally up your results and look at the organ or gland correlation. If you have several points in all or even one of the areas, you need to get that area under control. Any of the glands, when fatigued or compromised, can sabotage your ability to lose weight and keep it off. Weight loss is almost certainly one of the chief obstacles strangling every facet of our existence and negatively impacting our society today. Unless something is done NOW, future generations will continue to be hindered. For example, 72 percent of those applying to the U.S. military today cannot pass the basic requirements, including physical fitness! This is alarming.

I have witnessed wonderful results in my practice just by focusing on improving the hypothalamus and pituitary foundation pillar of hormonal health. I consistently see patients that come into the office who are under stress and have signals of diminished pituitary function. The hair analysis, symptom survey form and thyroid function tests, including the TSH values, have been effective tools helping me monitor and improve body function for my patients. We have had patients who have never before lost weight see the weight melt away because supplementation and lifestyle modifications create normal function of the brain-to-body mechanism. The mechanism in the brain is capable of sending the messages that the body needs to function optimally.[2]

CURBING YOUR DESIRE FOR SWEETS

Curbing your desire for sugar can be a HUGE challenge. Those small delicious morsels have an accumulative effect that tends to settle in the buttocks and thigh region in both men and women. I generally have to supplement my patients' desire for sweet foods. I highly encourage taking a whole-food chromium (up to nine tablets daily), as chromium helps cool the fire of desire or craving for sugar. Also, taking up to three caplets of the herb Gymnema a day will diminish the taste for sweets. I also recommend a whole-food bile salt, which also helps take away the passion for sweets. The best protocol I have found for bile salt usage is to take one tablet on the first day, then two on the next day, then three on the third day. Spread them over your large fatty meals. On day four, go back to one tablet and repeat the steps, increasing by one tablet a day until you reach three, then start over again. You don't want to alter the loop feedback mechanism and have your liver shut down its making of bile because you are supplementing too much.

FOR LONG-TERM SUCCESS

I want to direct you to Chapter 8 on liver function, where you need to follow the recommendations to achieve optimal detoxification and health. It is imperative that you follow everything suggested there, as this will be key for long-term success in maintaining your ideal weight.

Additionally for long-term success, you will want to monitor your saliva pH. Those who are acidic tend to be more toxic with a greater burden on their whole system, which will postpone weight loss. This can be an issue for many, as it is easy to stay in an acidic state since, as you've learned, normal cell metabolism and stress create an acidic condition.

The glycemic value of food also needs to be considered for long-term weight management. You can find a glycemic guide using any Internet search engine. I have included one in Chapter 16 as well. Focus on foods in the 50 to 80 range on the glycemic index. Important to keep in mind, though, is that even if the foods you consume are in the mid range, you don't want to go overboard and eat a lot. They still have calories. I would avoid the foods in the higher range because they will stimulate insulin release, which is the last fire you want turned on if you're trying to reach or stay at your ideal weight.

Taking flax oil, at one tablespoon per 100 pounds of body weight, and avoiding foods that cause inflammation—like sugar, dairy and trans fat—will assist your body in staying at a healthier state. Inflammation that can be detected by the "Dr. Bob's squeeze the wrist" test described in an earlier chapter. In addition to whole-body toxicity, having a boggy or spongy wrist usually suggests that the intestines, specifically, may be acting like a sieve, with undigested protein particles flowing through them. This creates havoc with the immune system and causes the whole body to be on alert, holding on to water to keep the particles in solution. I also suggest to my patients to use coconut oil as a way to cook, as it feeds the hormone circuit and helps you control the fire that burns the fat tissue. It can also be used as a replacement for butter.

REACH AND MAINTAIN YOUR NORMAL WEIGHT – ACTION STEPS

☐ For one week, journal what you are eating; do not go back and look at the week and give yourself the excuse that it was a "bad" week. Be brutally honest—you should be able to see the factors causing weight gain.

☐ Get into your birthday suit and look in the mirror. What do you see? Do you like the "man in the mirror"? Can you identify your body type?

☐ What does your physique look like? Is your belly way out? Do you like soda, beer, wine and other alcohol? If you do, how about cutting back?

☐ Take the quiz. What are your results?

☐ Based on the recommendations in this chapter, what tests should you have done to assess your current level of health? I suggest requesting TSH, T3, T4, urine iodine level and vitamin D tests.

☐ Start an exercise program. In my observation, there is a difference between exercise and recreation; jogging, running, rowing, biking that raises your heart rate and creates a real sweat is more effective for losing weight than are golf and bowling.

☐ Avoid refined grains, goodies, sodas and sugars. You can lose 10 to 15 pounds the first month just by saying no to soda—diet or original.

NOTES_____

7

THE TRUTH ABOUT TRANS FAT

Here we are at last, talking about the nitty-gritty when it comes to trans fat—a leading factor causing your pain, weight gain, reduced sex drive, high cholesterol and heart challenges! Well, it all started when scientists discovered that adding hydrogen at high temperatures to vegetable oil with the use of various catalysts would change the chemical property, bonds or hand-holding, of fat molecules and atoms. Saturated fat, one held hand or single bond, is generally hard and stiff at room temperature and can be heated without major change in configuration. Monounsaturated fat is one pair of held hands, or single double bond, and has more pliability and fluidity at room temperature. It is firm in cold temperatures and can tolerate a moderate amount of heat. Polyunsaturated fats, such as flax oil, with multiple pairs of held hands, are the most fragile and need to be kept cold, where they will still retain their liquid form.

A few points to add to your understanding are that hydrogen and oxygen are also a part of the molecular structure of the fatty acid chains. Polyunsaturated fats are pliable and tend to bend on themselves or appear in a C or cis position. When the heat and hydrogen are added to the vegetable oil at high temperatures, **there is a flip of one of the hands,** like twisting your wrist backwards, to add the hydrogen. **This results in a T configuration, or trans configuration, of the molecular shape.** This also changes the consistency of the formerly liquid oil to a firmer substance, which has been marketed to the masses as "butter without cholesterol." **The new substance, called "oleo" or "margarine,"** is now a saturated trans fat—**and all manmade trans fats are terrible for you!**

Your body uses fats in the creation of cell membranes. Every cell in your body has fat in it. The problem with trans fat is that its T confuses the system. Regardless of who you are, trans fat is not health promoting. The deal is, you cannot get away with fooling Mother Nature for very long. The body will start to respond and react and, over time, break down. Trans fat, please recall, interferes with your body's production of PG1 and PG3, the pain-relieving prostaglandins. You need more of those to balance the pain-causing PG2, which is stimulated or enhanced by trans fat.

Producing parts for repair and function requires time, just like making a luscious meal. The time frame I have brought to your attention so far is the half-life of trans fat. **The time to synthesize and process the manmade mutation is 51 days. That means that three months after you consume trans fat, you're still dealing with it.** Now, I also want you to be aware that the half-life of cis fat, or the good polyunsaturated fat, is 18 days. This means that this essential fat takes 18 days to be properly processed into cell membranes and have an effect on the body. I'm sure that tidbit of information is not making you do cartwheels either! But the significance is that when I make suggestions to my patients about health issues that are related to function dependent on fat, like hot flashes, ADHD, headaches, skin rashes and so on, I tell them to be patient—an uncommon American virtue. **It will take a minimum of 18 days to start seeing results.** I've witnessed it time and again: three weeks into the protocol and BANG!—the fat kicks in and patients see the beginning of health restoration.

As a side note, I normally tell patients that if they deviate from their diet by eating foods with trans fat, they should take a marine oil from a non-toxic source in capsule or liquid form at night to counteract the drain on healthy tissue-supporting fat reserves. Marine oil (I recommend anchovy and sardine oil) is a direct source of DHA and EPA. By now it should be pretty clear how people can consume a diet that either causes or relieves pain. Got it?!

Five percent of fats found in nature can be classified as trans fats. They occur naturally in the digestive system of ruminant animals, such as cows, sheep and goats. Some trans fatty acids are therefore present in meat, milk and other dairy products. These are mostly C18 monounsaturated trans fatty acids. Prior to the massive amount of trans fat now found in the diet, these C18 fats were used for energy. However, now that there is so much trans fat in our bodies, the C18 fats are incorporated into cell membranes with the potential to create major sickness and even genetic mutations. Without eating all the junk food "trans fat," and unless you overdose on the naturally occurring C18 trans fat, your body generally will use the C18 fat for energy and not cell membrane or tissue repair. Because so many people, especially younger people, consume more trans fat than the polyunsaturated cis fat, it is no wonder we have so many health ailments at younger and younger ages these days.

HYDROGENATION

Finally, let me throw one more little piece of information at you. I have been purposely using the term "trans fat," trying to keep it simple by not calling it by its other name, "hydrogenated fat" or "partially hydrogenated fat." Here is the bomb: The process of changing or hydrogenating fat, if carried out to the fullest, will result in a product that is firm and hard and not necessarily suited for a wide spectrum of use. Partial hydrogenation is when the process is stopped prematurely before complete hydrogenation occurs.

Food manufacturers prefer partially hydrogenated fat. Now, from all that I have observed over time, no one really knows what is created in the partial hydrogenation process. At least it won't be on the front page of any health magazine or journal. The travesty is, we have had an unsuspecting public, focused on "cholesterol free" for so long, that convincing them of the dangers of partial hydrogenation will be a monumental task. Then to add insult to injury, the facts are now being released that trans fat actually raises the level of LDL cholesterol and lowers HDL cholesterol—exactly the opposite of what it was touted to do. Trans fat, you'll remember, originated from a vegetable source without the supposed negative effects of cholesterol and fat found in butter—but, over time, the scientific community has finally realized it is worse than what it was originally going to improve or replace. If that doesn't grab you in the throat, I don't know what will.

When reviewing the LDL/HDL issue with the ALA pathway and linoleic pathway, you find that trans fat will raise the LDL level because it is sabotaging the body's ability to reduce inflammation by stopping the pain-relieving PG3. This is the body's way of compensating. THE BODY IS TRYING TO SAVE ITSELF. On the other hand, an inflamed and poorly functioning body needs to keep the HDL level low because its job is to take cholesterol out of vessels, but it needs that cholesterol at the site of inflammation. I have used chromium in my practice for patients to reduce the craving for sugar, which indirectly resets the HDL to naturally do its job, because with less sugar and reduced inflammation is a reduced need for LDL cholesterol.

SUMMARY OF TRANS FAT

- [ ] Cholesterol and saturated fat are suspected to be the primary cause of heart disease.

- [ ] Heated vegetable oil has been the alternative to butter and marketed as safe, but it is not.

- [ ] Heating vegetable oil alters the consistency and property of the molecules, confusing the body.

- [ ] The body uses fat to make cell membranes. Manmade trans fat is not compatible for human function.

- [ ] Trans fat causes pain and inflammation and interferes with the formation of PG1 and PG3.

- [ ] Partially hydrogenated fat is a dirty bomb with negative residuals.

- [ ] Sugar is the leading cause of inflammation, causing the body to compensate with elevated LDL cholesterol to put the inflammation fire out.

- [ ] Trans fat also causes inflammation, by increasing PG2 and inhibiting PG1 and PG3.

FOODS WITH NO TRANS FAT

Despite the ever growing tide of fast foods and convenience items purchased at the new American grocery store—aka service stations and corner franchise junk food "mini-marts"—it is possible to enjoy a diet that is free from trans fat. But having no plan is a plan to fail. Do you remember when you played sports—endless hours in the weight room, studying films, running through drills, sprinting until you thought you would upchuck your last meal? Well, I need to be your coach now—and for you military personnel and retired athletes that means I am blowing the "game face" whistle to get your attention! NO TRANS FAT!

I want you to use this next section as your playbook. So put on your smiling game face, and recall for a moment how all the practice you did before the big game or event always paid off, and as much as you didn't want to admit it on game day, coach was always right. Well, I am right in what I am about to tell you. Therefore, slowly read through the recommendations that follow because, quite honestly—and I am being real now—men are my toughest patients unless you do something different. No matter how big or little you change, it may seem like you will be exactly the same person, but that's not the case. Stop and re-read that! A fool is someone who repeats the same action over and over and expects a different result! You are going to actually need to go into a store and look around, avoid boxed items and buy real food that you can touch, smell, taste and squeeze. I want you to go slow when you shop—you may want a friend to go with you.

Breakfast Suggestions

Breakfast can come from any source other than from a package, a can, an envelope, a tub, etc. Breakfast will affect your insulin levels, which makes a major impact on your craving for sugar. Therefore, you should avoid starting the day with sweets, syrups or packaged foods. Rotating foods is important as well.

So where do you start? Avoid bananas, dates, figs, grapes and raisins in the morning. These foods will raise insulin and cause blood sugar variations and can affect the production of prostaglandins. Use wholesome non-sugar breakfast cereals (try rice cereals) with coconut milk, rice milk or almond milk. Greek yogurt is an option with cereal, but some do contain evaporated cane juice, which is another variation of sugar. You could bake a coconut. (Drill holes to let the milk out; cook at 325° for 10 minutes—mmmmmm good!) Don't limit yourself to traditional breakfast choices. Here are some suggestions for you to try:

Oatmeal (gluten free) is a simple food. It takes less than seven minutes to prepare. Boil water; add the oats and sprinkle with Celtic Sea Salt® and possibly some homemade applesauce. You can add almonds or sesame seeds, great sources of calcium. Walnuts and pecans are excellent sources of omega-3 fats. Any other seeds that you like can be added.

Rice cakes with almond butter, sesame butter or cashew butter are great options. Try no-sugar-added jellies and jams. Rice cakes do have a higher glycemic index, so take note if blood sugar levels are an issue with you.

Multi-grain pancakes made with water, coconut milk, rice milk or almond milk are another option. Spread with jelly containing no sugar. Kids love these with applesauce and cinnamon. You could even try REAL maple syrup (see Chapter 16 on sweeteners).

Breakfast cereals (gluten free) with no hydrogenated oils or sugar make a great option, too.

Organic eggs are an excellent source of protein and sulfur that is important for the production of collagen in the body. I am going to tell you, your cholesterol is not going up because of the egg, it is all the sweets, donuts, trans fat and sugar, plus stress. So sell the bass boat and cottage and stop eating the crap!

Gluten-free bread: If wheat gluten causes digestive challenges for you, try a sprouted grain bread like Ezekiel Bread or spelt bread with reduced amounts of gluten. You can find these options and others in the freezer section at your local whole-foods market. Or make your own bread!

Minimal to no dairy is best since cow's milk can alter the digestion of omega-3 fats. We tend to overeat dairy products, which can cause chronic ear infections leading to prescriptions of antibiotics, something we need to avoid.

Yogurt made from goat milk is a good protein source. Unfortunately, it is hard to find yogurt without added sugars or cane juice. You can sweeten plain yogurt with a few raisins, cinnamon or even crushed almonds.

Cheese: I would encourage you to use rice cheese. It is possible to buy pre-wrapped slices of rice cheese in a variety of flavors. Goat cheese, chevre and feta are great options and do not have the same inherent allergic issues to you as a human as cow's milk does. You can keep it in the refrigerator in olive oil and even infuse it with flavors like herbs and sun-dried tomatoes.

Squash can be eaten for breakfast! Cut whatever squash you like (I like acorn and butternut squash) into pieces for quicker baking time, place it in a covered glass dish and bake at 325° to 350° Fahrenheit. You can add cinnamon and organic butter when it is done (usually fork tender, about 45 minutes) and the whole family will like it.

Juice: I recommend *against* consuming orange and grapefruit juices when the weather is below 60° Fahrenheit, as these can cause mucus formation leading to congestion. Your best bet is apple juice or pure cranberry juice, diluted. I also recommend purchasing a juicer. I use a Vitamix® and juice beets, carrots, apples, cucumbers and a small piece of ginger. To get the maximum benefit of vitamins and enzymes, drink it right after it is made; do not save it and drink it later. Limit your serving size to eight ounces and eat some almonds or walnuts after the juice to slow down the potential insulin spike.

Water should be purified or from a quality spring. Check labels and research on the Internet, as some bottled waters are nothing more than tap water.

Meats should be organic. You don't want to consume the antibiotics or growth hormones that are given to animals and are still in their flesh.

Pork is not the other white meat. Whatever the pig eats, you eat. They wallow in mud among other materials and eat anything, healthy and toxic alike!

Seafood should be from clean sources; deep ocean fish are the best. I highly recommend *against* eating farm-raised fish. I would also avoid bottom feeders like shrimp and lobster. No deep fried fish; bake or broil only.

Lunch Suggestions

Packing lunches is an important part of maintaining a healthy lifestyle. This way you control what you and your family are eating. You can purchase antibiotic-free and nitrate-free lunch meats from whole-foods markets and from many grocery store chains. I buy antibiotic-free and nitrate-free turkey from the health food store.

You can substitute almond butter and jelly for the ole stand-by PB&J. Peanuts very often contain molds and yeast, which can cause immune issues. Almond butter is a much better choice. Vary the jelly, but just be sure it contains no added sugar. Vary your breads as well and stick to whole grains—gluten free may be best for you. (If you bloat with wheat products, it may be due to gluten sensitivity. I have, by the way, witnessed patients release 20 to 25 pounds by dropping gluten from their diets.) And, of course, no snack foods cooked in or containing hydrogenated fats! Instead, choose ones made with olive, safflower or sunflower oil. And remember that even these need to be eaten in moderation.

Build from scratch—meaning avoid "store prepared" (they have a lot of unfriendly additives)—veggie salads, tuna salad, egg salad, turkey salad, chicken salad sandwiches with rice cheese, lettuce and safflower mayo or whatever condiment you prefer. Use rice cheese pizza, pizza bagels, almond butter on celery and other fresh cut-up veggies. Make rice pasta with butter or nut milk in a container that keeps the contents warm.

Keep an eye on the condiments and avoid those with sugar or evaporated cane juice. Most condiments today, including the major commercial brands, always seem to contain sugar hidden as organic evaporated cane juice crystals. Condiments containing no sugar or corn syrup are best purchased from a health food store. **As always, you must read the labels!**

Finally, NO French fries cooked with partially hydrogenated fats!

Dinner Suggestions

Dinner is a very interesting meal. Families today rarely unite at the kitchen table for dinner as they have in the past. It is estimated that more than one-half of meals are eaten out of the home, including dinner. Part of the reason is the time it takes to prepare, cook and clean. But not having you or your family on medication for allergies should be reason enough to justify the additional time spent on food preparation and cleanup. You see, I have discovered over time—and this goes back to the "squeeze your wrist" test discussed in earlier chapters—that undigested food particles in the intestines that create the boggy wrist also create the same breakdown that causes chronic allergies. Dairy and peanut products are the two worst culprits.

I recommend having a family meeting to decide together what type of food you would like for your evening meals. Make it a fun, cooperative event where everyone participates, creating a unit for discussion and laughter. When everyone has a say in the matter, they are much more likely to go with the program.

As for my guidelines for good dinner choices, you can eat anything you want *except* for pork, hydrogenated fat, pre-packaged/powdered/boxed or canned food that contains preservatives and/or artificial colorings, flavorings, etc. My family does eat meat (normally organic, antibiotic-free), but you do not have to have red meat with every meal. We utilize rice pastas and, on occasion, fresh whole grain (versus the dried noodle version), beans, legumes and a variety of casseroles.

I am encouraging you to purchase as much food as you can fresh. Therefore, after you are finished with a meal, instead of having it as a leftover, you could freeze it and have it at another time. It's a great idea to pre-bake several meals prior to the beginning of the week. An enormous variety of foods can be used, such as squashes, zucchini, eggplant, potatoes, yams as well as different casseroles. The key is to make your food from scratch!

The great coach Vince Lombardi at one time was so upset with his Green Bay Packers that he sat them down in the locker room with a football in hand and said, "This is a football." I am sure he had special vernacular and adjectives that impacted his team forever as they went on to be one of great American football dynasties for that era. Well, your coach Dr. Bob is right in front of you now with a fresh head of vibrant green broccoli saying, "Gentlemen, this food, prepared raw, steamed, baked, mashed or roasted, has the potential to save your life. Eat it often." Remember, estrogen is at toxic levels in our environment today and will torpedo all your attempts to get and be healthy. Broccoli is one of the best food choices to control the negative impact on your delicate hormonal system. Pass this information on to everyone you know—we are all in the Super Bowl of life.

Your ethnic background and food taste will determine the type of foods you like to eat. Whatever your cultural preferences, your goal should be fresh, organic and alive food. BE CREATIVE! As I've been saying, varying foods is important. In our household, we use different organic tomato-based sauces and organic starter-type foods (organic broths). You could find some of Grandma's old recipes and use them; just be cautious of the amount of sugar they call for. I also encourage you to visit a bookstore, health food store and even the Internet for favorite recipes to utilize. There are many wonderful health magazines that have numerous recipes.

Salmon, tuna, eggs and chicken can all be used. There is even turkey/duck bacon, turkey/chicken sausage, lamb sausage and other alternatives, but remember to read labels because some of those products contain unhealthy oils, sugar and preservatives. Canned and pre-packaged foods are often mineral-depleting, metabolism-altering, toxin-creating chemical time bombs.

Sweet Suggestions

In case you didn't know this, you don't need dessert! I'm not exactly sure where this habit started; however, ending a meal with sugar puts enormous stress on the liver, pancreas and digestive system. Your body is busy breaking down proteins, and adding simple carbohydrates in the form of desserts can confuse things—this results in poor food combining with incomplete digestion and distress. It causes an enormous overload on the pancreas. Protein that is not digested properly putrefies, carbohydrates ferment and fats become rancid—all as part of the normal digestive process.

Desserts are nice on *special occasions*. They should be enjoyed sparingly rather than as a daily or even weekly indulgence. If you're going to have a dessert, use a recipe from a wholesome dessert book. There are also sources of naturally made cookies and desserts that can be purchased at your local health food store.

Some healthy dessert alternatives include using amaranth, an ancient flour product, in place of wheat. There are also healthy nut and grain ice creams. One of our family favorites is an apple crisp with non-dairy ice cream. There is a delicious coconut milk ice cream that I know you will enjoy. Or you can create your own home-churned ice cream made with organic-sourced cream (but, remember, special occasions only!). We get rave reviews whenever we bring the apple crisp to somebody else's house. Look at Chapter 16 on sweets for more on sugar options.

Snacks

I encourage you to consume a minimum of one apple, one carrot and a quart of water per day along with your other food choices. Having wholesome homemade snacks is ideal. Keep cut-up vegetables and fruits (as I've mentioned, pears, plums and apples are best) on hand for yourself and your family. Consume fruits only on an empty stomach, not after a meal.

Vary your snacks. There are healthy snack foods available without partially hydrogenated fats, including cookies without sugar. Popcorn made with olive or rice oil or an air popper is excellent. There is an assortment of rice crackers available; rice products are a pretty safe alternative for most people.

Visit health food stores and look into a food co-op. You can find excellent baking mixes that have very simple, wholesome ingredients. Have your children bake with you. This is a great wintertime activity.

COST OF FOOD

Consider, for a moment, your cost of over-the-counter medications— antacids, sinus medications and pain killers—for treating symptoms caused by improper eating. Eating healthier will drastically reduce money spent stocking your medicine cabinets. Did you know that 25 percent of our youth under 20 years old are on some type of prescription medication? That's staggering . . . and expensive.

I often hear people complain that it costs too much to eat healthy. But today many health food and conventional stores have competitive pricing. The cost for organic food may be slightly higher than conventionally prepared food due to supply and demand. I have found that prices in health food stores are usually lower in the second part of the month. Do your best to buy food on sale. Also, European, Asian and hometown family grocery stores carry wonderful and healthy foods at a price far lower than health food stores. For example, we have an Italian deli and bakery in our area that stocks a variety of healthy "old world" whole foods. And, in addition to providing healthy choices, a food co-op can save you hundreds of dollars every month. Find local food producers, such as farmer's markets. During harvest time, you can freeze many of the foods.

Yes, living healthy requires some work and participation, but the benefits are well worth the effort. Compare how much money you spend every time you eat out versus making that same food at home. Although it takes time, remember we need to spend more time with each other to cultivate meaningful relationships and emotional connections.

THE TRUTH ABOUT TRANS FAT – ACTION STEPS

☐ Read labels, and don't be fooled by items that say, "0 Grams Trans Fat" on the packaging. Instead, look at the Nutrition Facts, and if it says, "partially hydrogenated oil" put the package down! It's just another name for trans fat.

☐ Focus on cold-pressed vegetable oils. I recommend flax oil at one tablespoon per 100 pounds of body weight. Use olive oil to sauté your veggies. Avoid soy oils. I personally do not use canola oil.

☐ Eat whole foods; avoid processed, packaged items.

☐ Avoid sugar, including sugar disguised as evaporated can juice or crystals.

☐ Replace cow's milk with unsweetened almond, coconut or rice milk.

☐ Do not start your day with a refined grain product, such as donuts and pastries.

8

THE LIVER: YOUR BODY'S FILTER

My hope for you as you read this book is that you're fully grasping what a wonderful and complex machine your body is. You're like a mega computer system made up of trillions of cells all working together for the good of the whole. The body is a unit made up of many parts, none of which is greater than any other. I'm reminded of this remarkable concept as I work with my patients each day. When one part suffers, it affects the function of the whole. And when one part is brought to health, the rest of the body benefits as well.

THE ROLE OF YOUR LIVER

Your liver is an amazing organ, responsible for thousands of vital functions—some you may know about and many, many others you don't. Your liver, for example, performs hundreds of processes involving your sex life. Yes, as I said, a very important organ as I am sure you'll agree! Take care of your liver and it will take care of you.

When the liver is overworked, there is commonly an abundance of unprocessed natural and synthetic estrogen. In women, these hormonal imbalances are responsible for breast tenderness and heavy menses. But, as we've discussed, estrogen can also accumulate in men, creating prostate challenges, including prostate enlargement. In addition, the liver is involved in storing blood and vitamins, processing hormones, releasing blood sugar and protein, destroying unwanted organisms, creating bile for fat metabolism, eliminating unwanted consumed and cellular debris and much more. When you eat toxic, processed foods, your liver rearranges the chemical structures and releases residual by-products through your urine, sweat, breath and colon.

There's a process that occurs in the liver called the P450 system, which neutralizes medications and toxic substances by binding them to proteins and sulfur and then flushing them from the body. When liver function is compromised, this normal filtering process decreases, commonly resulting in degenerative conditions, including cancer and arthritis. Imagine driving through an expanding community with a limited sewer system. You'd likely smell the backup of sewage. Decreased liver function can be recognized in much the same way: foul breath, rank-smelling stool, skin rashes and skin tags (these are usually brown flarings off your skin).

An overworked liver places additional stress on the kidneys, which also aid in detoxification and can be considered the liver's "helpers." Symptoms of kidney stress include high blood pressure, swollen legs and general swelling of the body. Low thyroid function and constipation may result in additional stress on the liver.

Decades of treating patients and studying texts have brought me to a rather curious conclusion about the liver: It's an organ that's affected by emotions. Have you recognized more road rage over the last few years, as I have? You may have even noticed that those same people who are driving recklessly have a burger and fries in their hand as they shake their fist at you! They're eating fast and furiously while honking the horn and yelling at everyone around them. It comes as no surprise that studies show eating in a distressed state creates digestion problems and liver distress. In these conditions, your liver is literally being jammed by your emotions while simultaneously attempting to rid your body of toxic processed foods.

You can see what a vital service the liver performs, including storing the fat-soluble vitamins A, D, E and K, which are important for all body functions. Did you know, for example, that if you do not eat enough carrots, a source of precursors of vitamin A, you can suffer with chronic skin challenges and even spots in front of your eyes and night vision challenges while driving? Striving for peak liver function should be one of your daily goals.

EATING RIGHT FOR OPTIMAL LIVER FUNCTION

I encourage you to become more aware of what you put in (and on) your body and its effect on your liver. Foods and beverages such as diet soft drinks, trans fat snack and convenience products, alcohol and prescription medications create liver distress. Your liver needs to clear those burdensome chemical toxins found in conventional, non-organic food so they don't hinder cellular function. Every bite of over-processed, nutrient-empty food needs to be neutralized and eliminated by your liver detoxification system. So, why make your liver's job even harder by feeding it toxins? Instead, your diet should be based on fresh, organic, whole foods, as these require very little assistance from the liver.

Start each day with a glass of warm water and a wedge of washed, organic lemon. Let the lemon soak in the water for a few minutes, then drink the liquid and eat the lemon pulp, discarding the rind. This technique is a great way to stimulate liver function and digestion. I also recommend eating at least half of a red apple daily, as well as one-third cup of fresh, organic beets, baked or raw and grated. Add at least five small baby carrots or a medium whole carrot each day for your eyes and skin—to consume what I call "Dr. Bob's ABCs." These power foods will help stimulate normal liver function.

SIGNS THAT YOUR LIVER IS OVERWORKED

The skin is a report card on how your liver is performing. You may have suffered from acne when you were a teenager, and it's not uncommon for adults to have acne breakouts through their 30s. Your skin is actually one of the largest organs in the body and is used to rid the body of unwanted substances. In my experience, skin challenges can almost always be traced to an overworked liver handling toxic food, beverages and even over-the-counter and prescription medications. Similarly, I have noticed that individuals who have trouble falling asleep at night if they have consumed a beverage, medication or food item with caffeine in it tend to have liver distress. This would coincide with someone who already had the body signals associated with a compromised liver.

Proper liver maintenance will eventually ease skin flare-ups, though it may continue to take several months and possibly even years for your complexion to become fully clear. One note I'd like to mention on the topic of liver and the skin: Do not waste your health dollars having skin tabs removed with laser treatments, especially the little tabs around your neck. They will come back! Instead, cure the problem at its cause—work on cleaning up your liver.

The liver is a component in the stabilization of blood sugar by signaling cells to either store excess glucose or release it for fuel. Eating a diet high in sugar upsets this balance. In addition, the liver works with the pancreas during digestion. The pancreas releases insulin and enzymes for metabolism. Sluggish liver function decreases bile production, leading to digestive distress and impaired fat and sugar metabolism. Another reason a diet high in sugar and processed foods is destructive is because these nutrient-deficient products place incredible strain on the liver and pancreas and greatly increase the incidence of diabetes. As men, we have an added incentive to do everything possible to avoid this disease, as diabetics historically suffer from erectile dysfunction in all its forms.

Compromised liver function can commonly be associated with high blood pressure and depression. What you eat can impact your emotions, just as your emotions can impact the function of organs and glands. Go back to Chapter 1 and review how the CEO or hypothalamus connects the physical and emotional portions of your body. I've discovered through experience that the right fat choices have everything to do with behavioral and emotional health. I supplement patients who are depressed with organic high lignan omega-3 flax oil. The flax oil provides the precursor nutrients needed for DHA in the brain; this fatty acid is one of the many nutrients required for optimal brain health. A happy brain controls a happy body! I have also recommended the amino acid tyrosine for our patients who have depression. I will be discussing tyrosine in Chapter 15 on the thyroid.

IF YOUR GALLBLADDER HAS BEEN REMOVED

Do you still have your gallbladder? Over half a million gallbladders are removed every year in America through cholecystectomy surgery. Your gallbladder stores bile, which acts like a dish detergent that breaks apart the fats you eat and keeps them from accumulating on blood vessel walls and the lining of organs. When your gallbladder is removed, you lose this sack of stored bile and have no backup source for those times when more fat needs to be processed. Decreased bile levels lead to an accumulation of fat in the colon, resulting in an anaerobic (decreased oxygen) environment that is hospitable to cancer. You often hear that eating "saturated fat" causes colon cancer; in reality, cancer patients often have deeper challenges in the form of decreased bile output due to compromised liver function. If you've had your gallbladder removed, you should add a whole-food bile salt to your diet indefinitely to remain healthy and combat cancer and heart disease.

TOXIC OVERLOAD

We are bombarded by manmade synthetic compounds daily. I have mentioned that these substances must be cleared by the liver for you to thrive physically. I am strongly encouraging you to become very perceptive of your environment and what you are putting in and on your body. We are at the point in our society where you can no longer stay passive about chemical exposure: To maintain your health, you must become knowledgeable and proactive. Label-reading is critical, but what you read may not be completely factual. According to Lindsey Galloway and Elizabeth Marglin in a 2008 article titled "Beauty with a Conscience" in *Natural Solutions* magazine: "Even products marketed as 'natural' can come packed with hormone disrupters, carcinogens, toxic by-products and heavy metals. In fact, the average person applies up to 150 chemicals through skin and body care daily."[1] It is very important for you to become enlightened on what products are safe. I suggest searching the American Cancer Society's web page on products that are carcinogenic.

Let's take it up one more very serious step: The water you are drinking may be hazardous to your health. Wow, that's a bold statement. The municipal drinking water in America has deteriorated exponentially as of late and, unfortunately, very few Americans appear to be aware of the significance. Some time ago, a report was released about pharmaceutical trace residues being detected in and around municipalities. It was reported that up to 46 million Americans are being affected by pharmaceuticals in their drinking water. Items found in the water included a cholesterol and nicotine derivative, and many communities found the anti-convulsant carbamazepine. Other communities have detected other pharmaceuticals, including a tranquilizer and a hormone. Recently, the Environmental Protection Agency (EPA) reported that between 5 million and 17 million Americans are exposed to perchlorate, a toxic rocket fuel ingredient, through their drinking water. In an effort to tighten the reins on this downwardly spiraling situation, the federal government announced that it will develop the first standard to limit the amount of perchlorate permitted in tap water. The EPA said it is also moving to regulate up to 16 toxic chemicals in drinking water that may be damaging to human health.[2] Adding further insult, the unsuspecting consumer may not realize that a good portion of vegetables used in the United States are grown in regions where water is taken from the Colorado River, which is a source of perchlorate from agricultural farming runoff.

I urge you, do not be duped by your community officials and manufacturers of these compounds that they are at safe levels. Insist that your local community test the water that is produced by the filtration plant. I would also suggest that you may want to purchase a reverse osmosis water purifier system for your home. There are many places that sell them; just be sure to buy from a local company that can also service your unit. Today there are many health food and natural stores that have filter units available that you can take your own bottles to have filled. And, of course, there are also companies that will deliver filtered water right to your home or office.

ESTROGEN OVERLOAD

One of the largest challenges I've discovered affecting men of all ages is the magnitude of xenohormones or synthetic estrogens ingested from the environment. These hormones are commonly found in polycarbonate, one of the plastics carrying the recycling number 7 symbol. The plastic is clear, tough and lightweight, making it ideal for everything from bulletproof glass to water bottles, dental sealants, plastic eating utensils and food storage containers. Bisphenol A, or BPA, a key component in polycarbonates, is also found in the epoxy resins lining the inside of food and beverage cans, which leak in small amounts into the food or water in the containers. In fact, the list of items containing xenohormones is nearly endless, including the dust in our homes and our air and water! They are even sprayed on the fairway and greens at your favorite golf course. Therefore, do not place the golf tee in your mouth after hitting the ball 250 yards or lay your cigarette or cigar down then put it back in your mouth. And do not wipe dirt or grass off your golf ball with your tongue!

What worries some scientists is that BPA is an estrogenic "mimic," activating the same receptors in the body that estrogen does. In fact, BPA was first studied in the 1930s as a synthetic estrogen for women. "BPA is the largest-volume endocrine-disrupting chemical in commerce," says BPA critic Frederick vom Saal, a biologist at the University of Missouri, Worldwide. More than 6 million pounds of BPA are manufactured every year and vom Saal is convinced that BPA causes a host of problems including breast and prostate cancer.[3]

You and your entire family are continuously and relentlessly bombarded with BPA in the form of canned foods, car exhaust, fingernail polish, aerosol sprays, paints, noxious vapor compounds released from carpets, wall paper and magazine ink, just to name a few. The physical results of exposure and resulting liver congestion include spider veins, hemorrhoids, varicose veins, skin tags and the elusive cherry hemangiomas. Surgical intervention to repair or remove the compromise occurring in the vessels and skin of your body does not change the real reason you are experiencing these cosmetic challenges; they are body signals of a more severe toxic compensation—your liver is congested! The sexual consequences are even more sobering: tender breasts and heavy menses in women, prostate swelling and cancer in men, accelerated secondary sexual characteristics in children, increased sexual appetites in young girls and effeminate tendencies in boys.

Unfortunately, I see many young men, as young as 5 to 15, who are struggling with the effects of increased estrogen—uncontrolled feminization and obesity. This hormone creates cellular proliferation (growth) in the body. The delicate balance of these hormones is upset by stress and an unhealthy diet and lifestyle, leading to estrogen dominance and saturation. It is not uncommon for young men to have enlarged prostate and breast tissues from the estrogen found in the food they eat, including soy products. Again, males should not consume soy.

It's time to evaluate what can be done to protect you and your family from toxic exposure. The next epidemic I see occurring is estrogen-induced cancers in men—prostate and breast.

Do You Have Too Much Estrogen?

Processing estrogen in men and women is another of the liver's functions, and B vitamins are a critical component in this process. Once again, sugar and stress are major culprits that deplete the body of B vitamins. Now you can see why many people are unknowingly sabotaging their liver function. The chart below lists common signs of B deficiencies. How many symptoms are you experiencing?

☐ Apprehension	☐ Insomnia	☐ Weakness
☐ Depression	☐ Hypochondria	☐ Anorexia
☐ Nervousness	☐ Tendency to cry without reason	☐ Distraction
☐ Irritability		☐ Confusion
☐ Noise sensitivity	☐ Anxiety	☐ Craving for sweets
☐ Acoustic hallucinations	☐ Forgetfulness	
	☐ Indigestion	☐ Neuralgia
☐ Headache	☐ Poor appetite	☐ Dizziness
☐ Morbid fears	☐ Feeling of dread	

If you marked five or more boxes, you should evaluate your diet to determine what foods are overworking your liver and causing the symptoms of estrogen overload. These symptoms can usually be improved with proper whole-food B vitamin supplementation.

How to Minimize Your Exposure to BPA

Avoid plastic containers made of polycarbonate (any bottle or container made of polycarbonate that has the recycling number 7 on the bottom). Be aware that number 7 can also appear on plastics not containing BPA. Since it's not always possible to tell the difference, you're better just to avoid them altogether. I personally use a stainless steel container. I'm also seeing more glass-lined water containers with a protective cover on the market today.

When possible, prepare or store food—especially hot foods and liquids—in glass, porcelain or stainless steel dishes or containers, rather than plastic.

If you have polycarbonate plastic containers, don't microwave them. The plastic is more likely to break down and release BPA when it's repeatedly heated at high temperatures.

Don't wash polycarbonate containers in the dishwasher. The detergent may break down the plastic, resulting in the release of BPA.

If you have a child, grandchild or infant in the household, use glass formula bottles or those free of BPA plastic. BornFree (www.newborn-free.com) is one of the first companies manufacturing them. This is very important for the health of your children and grandchildren.

When possible, replace canned foods with fresh, frozen or foods packaged in aseptic (shelf-stable) boxes. Be mindful and look for "BPA Free" labels.

Currently, a possible alternative to polycarbonate is polyethylene terephthalate (PETE), which is marked with the recycling number 1 symbol, though there is no evidence that this is safer for you. You are always further ahead by using glass containers for your beverages.

Avoid older versions of Delton dental sealant. Dental sealants are plastic resins a dentist bonds into the grooves of the chewing surface of teeth to help prevent cavities.

The liver is just one organ in an amazingly complex machine, but it's a very critical one! Decreased function results in symptoms affecting almost every system in the body. The good news is that choices made to improve liver health ultimately benefit every other part as well.

YOUR BODY'S FILTER – ACTION STEPS

☐ Avoid processed foods, which stress the liver. Instead, eat organic, fresh, lightly steamed, raw or sautéed whole foods. This one step alone will assist in your whole-body detoxification. If you follow this pattern, special herbs or other cleansing products won't be necessary. Just heed the age-old advice, "Let food be your medicine and medicine be your food."

☐ Avoid items that may create an extra burden on liver function: medications, alcohol, soft drinks and artificial sweeteners or preservatives.

☐ To avoid estrogen-fed animal tissue, consume only organic meat products.

☐ Read bar codes on everything you buy for consumption! This may sound extreme, but some important information can be found there. The simplest marker is to look at the numbers under the bar code. Regardless of what country the food comes from, a code number starting with 8 means the product is from a genetically modified source; 9 means organic; all other numbers are considered standard or conventional—which means anything can be on them and they are not organic.

☐ Minimize your exposure to BPA by avoiding canned foods and by drinking water that has been bottled in glass containers instead of plastic.

☐ Eat Dr. Bob's ABCs daily: half a red apple, one-third cup of beets and four or five baby carrots.

☐ Avoid the constipation that leads to liver distress, by drinking more water and eating whole foods.

NOTES

9

HOW TO PREVENT CANCER

There are basic principles to healthy living, which, if *not* followed, will result in sickness and disease. In his book *The Answer to Cancer*, Dr. Hari Sharma states, "What, after all, causes cancer in the first place? Some tiny little thing in the tiny little cell causes the DNA to forget itself and become confused. Toxins cause cancer."[1] *Preventing* cancer is all about preserving and strengthening cellular intelligence.

The American Institute for Cancer Research (AICR) has reported, "Research has shown that most cancers can be prevented. Scientists now estimate that 60 to 70 percent of cancers are preventable through currently available information and simple changes in diet and lifestyle."[2]

The Western way of thinking is that early detection is the best way to stop cancer. But early detection leads to surgery, chemotherapy and radiation *after* cancer has already invaded the body. These treatments are reactive rather than proactive. Medicine attacks the symptoms but does not eliminate the cause. The treatments do not have anything to do with out-of-control DNA. In fact, drugs often weaken the immune system, creating an environment for more disease to appear.

Getting to the root of the problem eliminates cancer from occurring in the first place. One-third of all cancers are related to smoking. Smoking depletes the body of vital nutrients required for optimal long-term health—smokers tend to have lower levels of vitamin C, minerals and sulfur and, therefore, from my clinical experience I believe have a greater potential to suffer with chronic infections.

In addition to smoking, there are numerous other risk factors for cancer. Being overweight increases your risk for getting cancer by 40 percent. As noted, much of today's drinking water is contaminated, and canned foods are exposed to an inner layer of plastic that increases estrogen, which can cause abnormal cell growth. Eating man-tampered food rather than eating nature-made food also increases your risk.

A MATTER OF LIFE OR DEATH

Are you being tricked by the food manufacturers into eating foods that cause cancer? Many people are, but you don't have to be one of them. Within these pages are facts, statistics, proven strategies and sound advice based on years of clinical experience. The government recently released the new standard of what we should be eating, and it was more of the same-old: veggies, fruits and whole grains. But, by the looks of the scene at the beach and shopping plazas, it does not seem that people are creating their eating patterns based on the government's recommendations. Are you? How does the man in the mirror look these days?

Our culture and society have changed dramatically over the past few years—speaking on the phone is out, texting is in. Full names of products and companies have been shaved to a letter or two. Gas prices have been up—then down. Economic stability has been taking a roller coaster ride and has reached the lowest point in three generations. And although many communities are turning "green," many more municipal water supplies have been saturated with pharmaceutical residue. Food processing and delivery has changed. It has gone so far out of control that the names of countries where the food is sourced from must be on the label. Outbreaks of contaminated foods have taken dozens of lives per outbreak. Cloned animal products are now in the marketplace. The hype about organisms on the hands has created a market based on fear that an unseen epidemic of "bugs" may be the cause of your low health.

Do you know that some food manufactures have mapped, through the use of human genome technology, the taste receptors on the tongue? Taste receptors can be turned off or on depending on what you eat. For the sake of profit margins, the consuming public can be potentially misled into desiring foods that may alter our normal cellular function. This is a significant change in how products are being presented to consumers.

You, and your body, may be ignorantly tricked into being passionately addicted to morsels that are creating additional stress on your entire detoxification and immune systems. I find it awful that we are being conned into what may result in our premature untimely death. This revelation is very significant. I am constantly reading, listening and viewing new information to support my patients and so that the often misinformed public can have the upper hand when it comes to their health.

PREVENTING CANCER HOT SPOTS IN MEN

Now, allow me to share some tips I have garnered in my experience in regard to cancer.

Prostate Cancer

PSA testing for prostate cancer has been suggested for all men for early detection, to prevent a major metastasis before symptoms force you to be checked. I have, unfortunately, witnessed many men have their prostates removed by an aggressive surgeon, crippling their urinary and sexual function. I can comfortably tell you that the PSA is just a screen; it is *not* a definitive reason to go under the knife. I would suggest that if you have elevated prostate levels, you should follow these steps:

1. Stop soy and canned food – too much estrogen.
2. Eat more broccoli – lowers estrogen.
3. Drink pure water – no chemical impurities.
4. Stop all fast foods – no fried foods at all.
5. Eat organic animal tissue – no chemical-laced conventional meats.
6. Stop the dairy – go with almond milk.
7. Have your vitamin D level tested – it should be 40.
8. Have your urine iodine level tested – ideally, you would like it to be 95 percent excreted.

Let's talk for a moment about this last item on the list. I have consistently lowered PSA levels in my patients with iodine and vitamin D. As I've mentioned, I personally take 12 mg of organic iodine a day. Iodine physiologically is used by all the cells in the body. In men, the testes and prostate need iodine. As discussed in Chapter 6, there are anti-iodine elements, called halides, that fall in the same column as iodine in the chemistry periodic chart. These are bromine, fluorine and chlorine. These three chemical saboteurs fill the receptor sites that would normally host iodine. Iodine not only has to compete with these three, but because of their abundance combined with so little iodine available, your body does not have a fighting chance. Most of the patients I see with prostate challenges have a passion for fast food and estrogen foods, conventional meat, canned food and dairy. I have discovered over time that my male patients with deficient iodine levels from eating and/or exposure to estrogens have swollen prostates, commonly called benign prostatic hypertrophy, or BPH for short.

So, how to supplement your iodine? If your urine iodine test reveals that you need more iodine, you'll want to start slowly. If you have been exposed to bromine (hot tubs), chlorine (shower and pools), fluorine (toothpaste, water, mouthwashes), you may notice when you start taking iodine that your body will dump these halides, resulting in flu-like symptoms of nausea, headache, skin rashes and a metal taste in your mouth. To avoid this, I recommend starting out with 6 mg a day for a week or two, then building up gradually over a number of additional weeks to 12 mg; you would do this by adding 3 to 6 mg at a time. If you are over 200 pounds, you may even want to go up to 24 mg a day. To determine the amount that is right for you, it is best to have your iodine and even serum thyroid levels tested. For more information, see Chapter 15 on the thyroid.

Colon Cancer

Colon cancer, which is one of the leading causes of death in men, can very easily be prevented by eating green fiber foods. I can only say this, if you want to be healthy and live a long, productive life without having premature and unnecessary surgeries, you would do best to put your chin up and eat your greens—mixed green salads, cucumbers, cabbage, kale, Brussels sprouts, cauliflower and the best food of all, broccoli. If veggies tend to bother you, it is because your pH or acid/alkaline balance tends to be acidic. Alkaline foods force your body to dump toxins, which may cause you to feel uncomfortable. Therefore, start with veggies that are steamed, sautéed or stir-fried in olive or rice oils. Raw veggies may be a bit too much for your system; warming them breaks the fiber down and improves digestion with reduced stress. Now, I know that only 25 percent of men eat enough veggies every day. To make it easy to get my daily veggies, I bring a bag of them with me to the office each day: carrot sticks, celery, cucumber, half an apple, colored bell peppers and small tomatoes. By the way, tomatoes are excellent for optimal prostate health. An ounce of prevention is worth a pound of cure, so eat your veggies—and I do *not* mean the number one American veggie, French fries.

BECOMING AWARE

If you accept what the profit-driven media spews forth and what food manufacturers present, you will end up like many around you— overweight, sick and unhappy. The next time you are in a shopping mall or restaurant, look around at the people. Are they fit and trim? Is their skin clear and smooth? Are they laughing and enjoying themselves? And the next time you are watching television, count how many commercials are selling a prescription or over-the-counter drug that guarantees to make you "feel better" or "relieve" this or that. Be honest—is the United States winning the war on obesity and sickness? I don't think so.

I recently viewed a program about cancer research. They are "so close—please continue to contribute and we will have the answer soon." In reality, instances of certain types of cancer have been reduced because proactive women have stopped taking drugs used to mask the symptoms of hormone function. Their own blinded-by-the-facts physicians would have continued to prescribe these medications if an independent study had not been released revealing the serious effects of the medications![3]

No one wants to be duped. But you will be unless you decide to take control of your future.

Case in Point

A former patient of mine who decided a few years ago to follow the traditional medical protocol to treat her breast cancer—versus following a "get to the cause" recommendation—visited me at the office. She recently had reconstructive surgery following a bilateral mastectomy. She expressed concern to me after her own research revealed that the drugs she was prescribed could cause severe complications—including causing cancer in other areas of her body. She did not want the cancer to return, of course, but she was not fully informed by her conventional, symptom-treating health care providers about all of her options.

Hello? While the example I'm using is of a woman's issue, this could be you. I am risking being bold here because this is life-threatening stuff! I have witnessed the same with men who have a history of prostate cancer; they have well-meaning physicians who notified them that they had elevated PSA levels, with swollen prostate glands. They want to take the prostate out, without any explanation of what caused the swelling in the first place. Maybe you have experienced this. Therefore, you always want to get multiple opinions, including from health care providers who have treated patients without medications and surgery. The conventional medical treatment is not the *only* answer . . . read on.

Fewer Cases as Older Women Turn from Hormone Therapy

According to the American Society of Clinical Oncology, the declining use of hormone therapy may have led to a drop in breast cancer. This announcement was one of the biggest cancer stories of 2007. Women began abandoning hormone therapy in 2002, after the Women's Health Initiative—one of the strongest national studies of its kind—found that using estrogen and progestin increases the risk of breast tumors.

A study in the *New England Journal of Medicine* found that annual incidence rates dropped about 9 percent from 2001 to 2004, beginning in mid-2002 and leveling off by mid-2003. Rates dropped only in women who were 50 or older—the age range most likely to use hormone therapy. The drop was also sharper in women whose tumors are fueled by estrogen. The study's author noted that it's possible that other factors, such as declining use of screening mammograms, may also have contributed to the drop in new cases.[4]

ACRYLAMIDE AND THE LYMPHATIC SYSTEM

It has been reported from a variety of sources the last couple of years and even in my local paper that an item common in snack foods consumed today is a cancer-causing agent—it's the chemical acrylamide. Acrylamide has been in the news before, but like so many pieces of information we are flooded with these days, it was brushed aside. Acrylamide residues are commonly found in fried foods, one of the most popular food categories Americans eat. As I've mentioned, the number one vegetable in America is the French fry—and it is loaded with acrylamide.

Cancer is not a condition that just creeps up on you; it is a condition that can be prevented by, in part, avoiding fried foods. Once your body processes the food eaten, the chyme is transported through the intestines and portions of it are also carried by the seldom-discussed lymphatic system. When an abundance of fat is consumed in the diet, the lymphatic system can become sluggish.

When I was writing the chapter on the lymphatic system for my book *Dr. Bob's Drugless Guide to Balance Female Hormones*, I realized that so many of our health challenges are due to toxins in the environment. Many people with poor health have livers that are so congested that the lymphatic system backs up, just like a sewer would. Because the lymph glands are swollen in advanced cases of

destructive conditions like cancer, the conventional medical think-
ers have the public convinced that the lymphatic system is "the bad
guy," but I can assure you it is not. The lymphatic system is doing the job it was designed to do: disposing of the toxins that have
entered your system, either by choice in what you've consumed
or by environmental exposure. The challenge is that the lymphatic
system is often overwhelmed with the massive amount of work
it needs to do. When cancer supposedly spreads to the lymphatic
system, in reality the lymph nodes are congested from attempting
to do everything they can to clear out the debris and invaders in the
form of bacteria, free radicals and cancer cells.

The lymphatic system has an enormous presence in the abdomen,
but it does not have the help of its own pump like the cardiovascular system does. My suggestion to you and to all of my patients
for getting the lymphatic system moving and draining is to create
a movement of the lymph fluid in what is a vacuum-like phenom-
enon for the lymph system. This particular strategy was revealed
to me by one of the massage therapists who practices in my office.
She noticed that when she would complete a full-body lymphatic
drainage massage, her female clients who'd had their lips fully covered with lip gloss or lipstick would magically see the lip makeup
get absorbed once their lymphatic system was activated. The lips
are connected to the lymphatic system, as are all other parts of the
body. When she activated the lymph system with the massage, the
lipstick was quickly absorbed. This same process happens every
time you apply any chemical on your body; it is absorbed and used
and eventually processed by the liver.

An excellent way to get the lymph moving is through exercise. I
suggest getting a large (55 cm) ball and sitting on it and bouncing
for two to three minutes a day. You could also get a mini-trampoline
and bounce. The movement from the ball and or mini-trampoline
literally pushes the clear lymph fluid through the lymph ducts.

Another key to keeping lymph moving is to drink water and avoid dairy, as dairy plugs up the lymph system.

You may notice flu-like systems at times when you drink a bit too much alcohol or if eating or drinking something that is out of the norm for you. The symptoms of nausea often can be a signal from the overworked lymph nodes in your abdomen, which are connected to the "second brain" or nervous system in your body called the enteric nervous system. The lymph system is sending messages up to the brain to your body's CEO, the hypothalamus, which is coordinating the reset of your system back to your "normal." In a nutshell, your lymphatic system is responsible for helping the rest of the body move out unwanted and overloaded toxins. To assist the lymph system in removing these toxins, I have had great success relieving patients' flu-like symptoms with the herb peppermint leaf. Peppermint leaf has many benefits: Not only does it promote liver and gallbladder function for removing toxins, but it is also anti-microbial, which helps prevent the flu.

A DRUGLESS APPROACH TO TREATING CANCER

The assessment of body saliva or blood serum pH, or the measure of acid/alkaline, is a state of physiology that is analogous to the acid (vinegar-like) or alkaline (baking soda–like) level in your body. *Cancer cells thrive in an acidic environment.* Cancer patients who have presented to my office for assessments are generally on the acidic side of the saliva test paper.

Oxygen Radical Absorbance Capacity, or ORAC, is a method that measures a food's ability to absorb free radicals. Free radicals irritate the body and tamper with cellular integrity. Smoking, alcohol and pollution increase the instance of free radicals. At the top of the list of foods with a high ORAC are organic red apples. Red apples provide vitamin C, which is an anti-cancer nutrient. Red apples decrease estrogen and keep blood sugar levels steady. Eating red apples also lowers cholesterol (sometimes as much as 13 percent) and keeps bile flowing—promoting a healthy alkaline balance.

I suggest eating half an apple, either warm or at room temperature, daily. Every two or three days, prepare a warmed half apple by cutting it into quarters and inserting a clove in each section. Place the two sections in pure water and heat on your stovetop. Discard the cloves and eat the apple segments. Apples provide essential minerals that make your body function optimally. You will notice improved bowel transit time by adding apple to your diet.

Let me remind you here about my "ABCs"—apples, beets, carrots. All three foods facilitate bile flow and function. Eat at least one-half of a red apple, one-third cup of grated raw or baked beets and four or five baby carrots every day. In addition to these ABCs, healthy people eat a variety of foods. Foods that promote health include organic brown rice, beans and nuts. As mentioned, cabbage, broccoli, cauliflower and Brussels sprouts protect your DNA and help in detoxifying your liver. You need not eat all of your veggies raw—they are also delicious lightly steamed or sautéed. Tomatoes are good for prostate issues, but nightshades—potatoes, eggplant, green peppers—can create liver distress symptoms when the liver has been overworked.

I have found that those patients who have digestive distress with onion, garlic, radishes and green peppers tend to have pasty thick bile with gallbladder distress. These are actually excellent foods, as you will see in Chapter 17 on the Page Diet, a template for eating the right food, but when your body is sluggish you will feel a bit queasy over the eyes with possible pain on the right lower ribs below the rib cage. You may notice a heavy metal taste in your mouth.

The four or five baby carrots per day provide vitamins for the liver, which is the storehouse for vitamins A, D, E and K. Eating greens will also give your body what it needs to thrive. Onions, garlic, chives and leeks contain allicin and sulfur, which equate to vibrant life by breaking down toxins. Garlic has been used for centuries as a natural antibiotic. Also, incorporate ginger into your meals. Ginger is an anti-cancer nutrient. Garlic and ginger are a power duo for the immune system.

So, what should you *not* eat or drink if you are dealing with cancer or if you are just hoping to avoid it? It's the same list that we have been discussing throughout this book. Fried foods can cause cancer. Wheat and soy deplete your body of essential zinc, which is critical for optimal health and healing at the basic cellular function for your prostate gland, pancreas and memory. Unless you have an orange tree in your backyard and squeeze your own, orange juice from the grocery store is man-tampered. Avoid eating cold leftovers; they are hard to digest and contain no vitality. Dairy can cause chronic pain. Avoiding cow's milk and ice cream will make a significant difference in eliminating body pain. I call donuts "torpedoes of death"—avoid them, and all pastries, especially for breakfast.

Your principal meal, by the way, should be lunch. This is so that the food will have time to digest and provide energy for your body. Eating after 7 p.m. is not recommended, as it causes the digestive system to stagnate.

HOW TO PREVENT CANCER – ACTION STEPS

☐ Get eight hours of sleep each night. Your body releases growth hormone at night, and growth hormones promote healing.

☐ Stop smoking.

☐ Avoid sugar. Cancer cells have a passion for sugar. The more insulin in the body, the more inflammation—and inflammation causes cancer.

☐ Start your day with a stewed apple and clove. Eating at least half of an apple a day creates energy in your body.

☐ Be happy! A positive attitude creates more of an alkaline pH in the body, while anger or sadness creates an acid pH.

☐ Don't eat when stressed or when you are driving, watching television, reading the newspaper or at your work desk; this alters your digestion and compromises all that the good food is designed to do and be.

☐ Eat fresh veggies. Vary them: raw, steamed and sautéed. Greens protect DNA.

☐ Stop frying meats and eating fried foods, including French fries. Frying creates heterocyclic amines or mutagens, which have been shown to cause cancer in animals.

☐ Take turmeric daily—one-fourth teaspoon with a meal. Turmeric is a great antioxidant that helps protect DNA. Turmeric inhibits leukemia, is anti-cancer, anti-bacterial, and anti-inflammatory.

☐ If you consume dairy, do it with nothing else. This will be better for digestion.

☐ Cancer cells love an acidic environment created by eating sugar, over-consuming protein and living with stress.

☐ Have your serum vitamin D and urine iodine levels assessed and then supplement accordingly. I suggest 2,000 IU to 10,000 IU of vitamin D_3 daily. And, as I've mentioned, I personally take 12 mg of organic iodine daily based on my TSH, T3 and T4 levels. We'll discuss this more in Chapter 15 on the thyroid.

☐ Minimize or balance acid ash foods, such as animal proteins, with alkaline foods, like broccoli, cabbage and cauliflower.

10

"MR. ED": MANAGING ERECTILE DYSFUNCTION

Just like every other system in the body, the male sex organs are an engineering masterpiece. Glands, hormones, muscle, tissue and blood are all designed to work in tandem and create one of the most amazing and wonderful sensations available to men. There is no greater feeling than the awesome rush of an ejaculation as you look into the eyes of your mate.

I wish every couple could experience this wonderfully intimate moment each time they desired sexual intimacy; unfortunately, many men (and many of their female partners!) are frustrated when male sex organs don't function as intended. The cause may be neglect or ignorance, but the result is the same: couples who are missing out on the exciting sexual relationship they should experience.

This chapter will cover the following male sexual dysfunctions I commonly see and treat in my practice:

- erectile dysfunction
- ejaculation dysfunction

- diabetes-related dysfunction
- pain syndromes
- Peyronie's disease
- condom use and unfulfilled intercourse

Most men feel uncomfortable discussing their sexual desires and dysfunction issues with their women; in fact, I often speak with women about their man's challenges long before I actually have a frank conversation with the man at all. I recently ran across an article in the *Wall Street Journal*'s Health Matters section entitled "Is Your Wife Pushing You to See a Doctor? Read This—and Go." The article continued: "Doctors say wives are in a unique position to persuade their husbands to seek medical care. Erectile function is an important barometer of a man's health."[1] I've discovered that women are usually more open, partly because they start talking about menstruation and sexuality in a clinical way early in their teens as puberty approaches. The conversation continues with their friends and spouse as they experience hormonal changes throughout their lifetime. In contrast, men's early sexual communication is likely to be locker room stories and boasting, which may or may not be factual. Men generally don't sit around discussing their challenges or inability to have sex, but these dysfunctions are deeply hurtful to a man's ego and sense of manhood. The inability to achieve a spontaneous erection during or before foreplay and penetration is like taking a weapon away from a soldier. A frank discussion of the problem—while absolutely necessary—takes trust, vulnerability, honesty and humility by all parties involved.

When patients want to talk to me about sexual concerns, they usually approach me the same way: With glassy eyes, they slowly lean forward and whisper, "Dr. Bob, I am having problems getting an erection," or, "Dr. Bob, I can get an erection . . . but I can't ejaculate." Quite often women will tell me the same thing about their husband or boyfriend. Some women tell me that their man wakes them up three or four times in the night going to the bathroom to urinate. Then there are men who don't desire sexual intimacy, who have pain that prevents them from performing or who won't give a reason for their lack of interest to their hurt, confused spouse. The good news is that there is hope! Let's look, in turn, at each of the dysfunctions listed above and find out why things go wrong and what can be done to solve the problem.

ERECTILE DYSFUNCTION

Erectile dysfunction is by far the most common sexual dilemma I treat in men. This includes the complete inability to achieve an erection and the inability to maintain an erection when one is present.[2] The clinical criterion to diagnose this dysfunction is when it occurs more than 25 percent of the time when you are aroused. It's been suggested that between 20 and up to 30 percent of men over 40 years of age suffer from erectile dysfunction. This is a staggering statistic and a symptom of the declining health of our population. It's also a relatively new term; you will not find "erectile dysfunction" in older medical text books. The word "impotence" was used for this condition until the pharmaceutical industry created a drug to treat erection challenges. "Impotence" had negative connotations and drug companies wanted to de-stigmatize the condition, so they made it more appealing by coining the term "erectile dysfunction" or "ED."

Erection challenges are a sign of the times and have become epidemic in our culture. As a result of poor diets filled with excessive processed convenience foods, lack of exercise and the increased use of stimulants, men have basically worn their bodies out. Increasingly, men are also exposed to estrogens in the water supply that are winding up there from the urine of patients consuming hormone replacement therapy or discarded medications that have been dumped in the toilet. When a patient finally reluctantly brings up the subject with a medical doctor, it's far easier for that doctor to write a prescription and treat the symptom than to coach the patient in lifestyle modifications that will treat the cause of ED. This is a modern Western cultural dilemma. Below is a list of common current conventional medical reasons for erectile dysfunction:

- diseases and conditions such as diabetes, high blood pressure, heart or thyroid conditions, poor circulation, low testosterone, depression and nerve damage from surgery

- pharmaceutical drugs such as blood pressure medications (beta blockers), heart medications (such as digoxin), some peptic ulcer medications, sleeping pills and antidepressants

- nicotine, alcohol[3] and cocaine

- stress, fear, anxiety and anger

- unrealistic sexual expectations that make intimacy a chore or task rather than a pleasure

- poor communication with your spouse or significant other

- a "vicious cycle" of doubt, failure or negative communications that reinforce the erection problem

COMMON DIETARY AND STRUCTURAL FACTORS PROMOTING ERECTILE DYSFUNCTION

- Diets high in wheat and soy products deplete zinc. Zinc is necessary for many enzyme reactions to occur in the body, including prostate health, memory, blood sugar stress (zinc helps make insulin for blood sugar handling) and tissue healing.

- Vegetarian diets high in copper are often low in zinc and contain inadequate complete proteins.

- Diets high in soy tend to add more estrogen factors, antagonizing testosterone. Young men raised today have been exposed to increased levels of estrogen from birth.

- Conventional meat and other products increase our exposure to estrogen compounds.

- Exposure to synthetic compounds, including medications and industrial compounds, create a gallbladder/liver burden.[4]

THE PHYSIOLOGY OF ERECTILE DYSFUNCTION

So, just how does the erection mechanism work? The autonomic nervous system is the major component responsible for erections. This system functions just like it sounds: automatically. What a brilliant design; we don't have to think about breathing, swallowing, having bowel movements and a whole host of other normal body functions that are necessary for life. This automatic system is divided into two major parts that work in unison with each other: the sympathetic and the parasympathetic nervous systems. Simply stated, the sympathetic system speeds you up, and the parasympathetic slows you down. Ideally, they are balanced to allow your body to work flawlessly. You can think of these nervous systems as the gas and the brake on a car; at times you need to accelerate and at other times you need to slow down.

Unfortunately, in most of the sexually compromised patients I treat, the sympathetic nervous system is on overdrive and dominates the parasympathetic. The reason this dominance is so destructive sexually is because the parasympathetic system is responsible for achieving and maintaining erections. Lowered parasympathetic activity leads to lowered erection function. Lowered erection function leads to diminished sexual activity. Diminished sexual activity leads to unhappy, frustrated, disconnected couples. You get the picture.

The sympathetic nervous system's dominance is commonly due to poor diet choices with too much sugar and artificial stimulants, lack of exercise, high levels of stress and no time to rest.

ERECTILE DYSFUNCTION DUE TO MISALIGNMENT

The parasympathetic nervous system has a direct connection from the brain to the penis by way of the vagus nerve. When the nerve is compressed, signals to achieve and/or maintain an erection are partially or fully blocked. These compressions, or subluxations, may occur in the neck where the nerve first exits the brain or in the lumbar or sacral area of the lower back where the message is delivered to the genitals. Daily events can precipitate subluxation: poor posture, poor sleep habits, motor vehicle accidents, stressful work conditions, exercise and sport injuries and gravity. With regular spinal adjustments, many of my patients suffering from ED have reported naturally occurring, consistent erections—without the use of medication.

Stimulation of the vagus nerve has also been used by conventional medical practitioners to decrease depression, creating an interesting correlation between erectile dysfunction and depression. While researching medical information for erection challenges, I discovered that some institutions are implanting vagus nerve stimulators to treat both depression and erectile issues. This strongly suggests an association between the nervous system, depression and erectile dysfunction.

If you are suffering with erection issues, you should have your lower pelvis and spine assessed and corrected accordingly before you consider taking any medication with serious side effects. I've had many smiling wives or girlfriends of my ED patients come to the office thanking us for improving their sex life while avoiding the negative side effects common with most erectile dysfunction drugs.

MEDICATION SIDE EFFECTS AND ERECTILE DYSFUNCTION

Erectile dysfunction is a side effect of many common drugs. For example, in a recent issue of *The Journal of Urology,* Kaiser Permanente

Southern California's director of research Steve Jacobsen reports that men who use non-steroidal anti-inflammatory drugs (NSAIDs) three times a day for more than three months are at a 22 percent increased risk of erectile dysfunction.[5] Three other significant and highly prescribed drugs that cause ED are beta blockers, antidepressants and statins. We'll discuss each of these in detail.

Beta Blockers

Beta blockers are used to treat high blood pressure, migraine headaches, anxiety, heart palpitations and glaucoma. These drugs interfere with the flow of blood to the penis by blocking the action of the chemical transmitters that communicate between nerves and other tissues.

High blood pressure is very common in the Western world, caused largely by a poor diet and stress. Weight is not always an accurate measure for who likely suffers from high blood pressure; I have seen very heavy individuals with normal pressure and thin folks with high blood pressure.

Today's pharmaceutical community continues to lower the numbers that are considered normal for blood pressure; I sense they are doing this to sell more medication. Before you treat with medication, try drugless methods to lower your blood pressure. First, make sure your diet is providing ample calcium. Do you get cold sores, leg cramps at night and colds easily? These are all signs of inadequate calcium. I encourage my patients to take calcium in the form of calcium citrate or lactate. Calcium helps relax the very tight blood vessels that may increase blood pressure. You could also incorporate kelp and black cohosh, two herbs with a history of naturally lowering blood pressure.

I have successfully helped many patients with blood pressure challenges by assessing and supporting vitamin D levels. Vitamin D impacts calcium absorption. Sunshine converts the cholesterol in your skin to vitamin D. Is it a wonder why we have such a variety of health issues in America? Staying out of the sun—that great ball of light that nature gives us as a way to lower cholesterol—does not promote optimal health. I encourage early morning and late afternoon sun exposure without toxic sunscreens—before 11 a.m. and then between 4 p.m. to 6 p.m. are good times to avoid getting burned. You do want to stay out of the sun during the hours of most intense exposure, between 11 a.m. and 3 p.m.

Eliminating refined grain, sweetened carbohydrates (pastries, donuts, muffins, etc.) from the diet is another natural treatment, because carbohydrates increase insulin, which causes sodium to be retained in the system and elevates blood pressure. Mung beans (commonly used to make bean sprouts) consumed daily are also a helpful remedy. Soak one tablespoon of Mung beans in hot water and drink the water. Add eight ounces of water back in the beans and repeat twice during the day. At the third session, drink the water and also eat the beans.[6]

Organic pomegranate juice is another natural blood pressure remedy. I recommend drinking two 1-ounce servings of a day. Additionally, increased water intake from a pure source results in thinning of the blood and lowered pressure. My patients have also experienced reduced blood pressure by using Celtic Sea Salt® and alfalfa tablets.

Antidepressants

Many of the new patients coming into my office suffering from erectile dysfunction are taking prescription medications for depression. The risk and severity of sexual side effects depends on the individual and the specific type and dose of antidepressant, but common sexual side effects include reduced sexual desire, erectile dysfunction and difficulty achieving orgasm or ejaculation. The most common antidepressant that my male patients discuss or have a history of taking is Zoloft®. My observations have been that 35- to 45-year-old high achievers are the most common users, followed by the "mid-life crisis" group who are getting depressed as they look at where they are in the scheme of life and score themselves low on their own report card of victories and defeats.

Many men suffer silently. I have been amazed to speak to very "together" looking and sounding men at social gatherings, only to later discover their difficulties when they become a patient of mine and "dump" on me all of their woes and pull out their laundry list of meds: blood pressure, cholesterol, digestive, sleeping aids and finally antidepressants. (I am now also beginning to see more medications for the pre-diabetic wave that is starting.) The group to be aware of, that impacts sexual ability more than the others, is the selective serotonin reuptake inhibitors (SSRIs)—Paxil®, Prozac® and Zoloft®. I have discovered that, both in men and women, inadequate omega-3 oil consumption, an overabundance of trans fat and subpar thyroid function, which will be discussed in Chapter 15, are the leading factors precipitating depression.

Exactly how these antidepressants interfere with sexual desire and function remains the subject of ongoing debate and investigation. Unconfirmed or unverified theories abound; for example, some blame the sedating effect of certain antidepressants for dampening sexual desire. Others speculate these antidepressants cause chemical changes in the parts of the brain regulating sexual desire and function. Complicating all of this is the effect of depression itself in decreasing sexual desire and function.

It's impossible to predict which individuals are most likely to develop sexual side effects while taking an antidepressant. In some cases, sexual side effects may improve once your body adjusts to the medication; but in other patients, sexual side effects may last for the duration of treatment. If you experience sexual side effects while taking an antidepressant, consider these strategies:

- Talk to your conventional doctor about the possibility of changing your dose of antidepressant medication.

- You may want to consider taking a medication requiring only a once-a-day dose, and schedule sexual activity before taking that dose if you are not in a position to discontinue antidepressant medications at this time.

- You should also contact an experienced natural health care provider for assistance with your diet. To get started on the right track with diet, be sure to read Chapter 17 of this book on the Page Fundamental Diet Plan.

- Consider having a thyroid test to determine whether there are other natural ways to treat your depression.

How well these strategies work depends on the specific drug and your individual circumstances. If sexual side effects are troublesome, talk to your doctor before discontinuing your medication. Conventional medical physicians are traditionally of the mindset that any approach other than the pharmaceutical protocol is unsafe. My experience indicates that if you are motivated to change your diet, exercise and take the supplements your body needs, you will be pleasantly surprised. You can be depression and antidepressant free!

Depression can be precipitated by many factors, including insufficient amounts of omega-3 oils that are found in foods such as flax oil, walnuts and greens. Consuming an abundance of snack or convenience foods with trans fat or partially hydrogenated oils is also problematic; trans fats, as you have learned, interfere with the production of DHA, a long-chain fat needed for optimal brain health and an element commonly deficient in depressed patients. I test my patients' DHA levels with a blood spot test and supplement accordingly. I have also witnessed depressed patients improve when their thyroid is assessed and supplemented with iodine and the amino acid tyrosine, and I have successfully treated depressed patients by including marine and animal proteins in their diet, especially turkey and tuna. I also encourage chicken thighs and legs (with healthy fat, which is beneficial for the brain) and adding whole-food B vitamins.

Of course, there are causes of depression that are purely psychological, such as poor self-image, stress, abuse, anger and un-forgiveness. If you suspect that your depression may have a psychological as well as physiological component, seek out a qualified counselor. There is no reason to suffer alone!

Statin Drugs

Statin drugs are marketed as a treatment for everything from lowering cholesterol to preventing cancer. These drugs have very chilling side effects that include erectile dysfunction and liver disease. They may also cause increased body pain and create a deficiency of coenzyme Q1O, an energy-creating powerful antioxidant. Statin drugs work by sabotaging cholesterol metabolism in the body. Cholesterol, as we've discussed, has a bad reputation because its role in human physiology is not well understood. In reality, cholesterol is neither good nor bad; it's a vital component in many important functions in the body, including the production of steroid hormones.[7]

Without cholesterol, your cell membranes won't function like they should and your adrenal glands will be unable to produce testosterone, progesterone, estrogen and cortisone. Cholesterol levels only become problematic when they are elevated; this is usually a result of cholesterol's normal response to inflammation in the body due to poor eating habits. Avoiding partially hydrogenated or trans fats and lowering sugar intake are helpful in controlling cholesterol levels. Tragically, the public has bought into low-fat/no-fat diet fads that are loaded with deadly manmade trans fats. For years, the medical community promoted these harmful diets and people were simply ignorant of the proper role of cholesterol in good health.[8] Eating an apple each day can lower your cholesterol 13 percent, and you can lower cholesterol 40 percent by adding beets to your diet.

TREATING ERECTILE DYSFUNCTION

After an assessment of ED is made, the first method of treatment should be spinal corrective care. Many patients respond quickly to spinal manipulation that restores proper nervous system function to their genitals.

Adrenal fatigue is the next culprit, which is treated by cutting sugar out of your diet. (As you will read in Chapter 13 on the adrenal glands, over-consumption of sugar stresses the adrenal glands' ability to make sex hormones and transmitters.) To stop the sugar craving, supplement with whole-food chromium, a mineral commonly deficient in those who crave sweets, and the herb Gymnema, which takes away the taste for sweets. Cutting out sugar is absolutely essential if you want to give your adrenal glands any possible chance of being restored. This includes sweet fruits such as bananas, raisins, grapes, pineapple and any dried fruit. (Pears, plums and apples, as I've mentioned, are an excellent fruit choice any day of the week.) You should also avoid energy drinks loaded with stimulants, as they too stress adrenal function.

And, as mentioned, zinc deficiencies are quite common in men with ED, causing enlargement of the prostate and frequent urination. Zinc plays a role in memory, the production of insulin, healing, the immune system and about 90 other functions. White spots on the fingernails are a common symptom of low zinc levels, as are large facial pores. In my office, we incorporate a zinc taste test and supplement with a liquid product accordingly, eventually changing to a dry tablet.[9] Wheat and soy should be avoided, as they tend to deplete the body of necessary zinc.

Iodine and tyrosine supplements are used when thyroid function is the cause of ED. There are also herbs available for treatment. The herb tribulus helps stimulate the body's ability to create testosterone, increasing libido. My patients also routinely take a maca root–based product along with tribulus. The combination has helped nearly every man I have suggested it to, to restore hormonal balance and increase function. These products can be purchased at **www.druglessdoctor.com**.

Finally, appropriate lifestyle modifications should be made. Herbs and supplements are beneficial, but the ultimate goal is to help the body function fully with whole foods and the elimination of toxic habits.

NOCTURNAL ERECTIONS

Before we move on to ejaculation dysfunction, let me mention something here about nocturnal erections. It's possible for a man to have three to five erections during the night, each one lasting up to 30 minutes. If you wake up in the middle of the night or in the morning with an erection, it means your body is functioning correctly. It may also be a sign that your daytime erectile dysfunction has psychological roots rather than physiological ones. The problem may be stress related, due to performance anxiety, or the result of relationship difficulties stemming from other issues. You may also experience difficulty getting an erection if you have recently ejaculated or have had multiple sexual encounters over a short period of time. You may desire to have sex, but your body has a refractory period during which it replenishes sperm and seminal fluid and the ability to achieve an erection is diminished. This is a normal part of the sexual cycle.

EJACULATION DYSFUNCTION

As we've discussed, the nervous systems that work in tandem are the parasympathetic (slows you down) and sympathetic (speeds you up). The parasympathetic system is in charge of achieving and maintaining erections, while the sympathetic nervous system is in charge of ejaculation. Because these functions are controlled by separate systems, it's completely possible to have one without the other. (A normal erection and the inability to ejaculate, or the ability to ejaculate with a very soft erection.) Optimally, the two systems are well balanced so that both erection and ejaculation can be achieved at the appropriate time. The adrenal glands release chemical transmitters that stimulate the sympathetic nervous system for ejaculation. These significant transmitters are generally low or depleted in individuals who experience ejaculation dysfunction.

To manage these challenges naturally, you should eliminate sugar from your diet, avoid processed foods, minimize stress and eat whole foods. Alcohol intake should be moderate and if you smoke, you should start a plan to quit immediately.

Another ejaculation dysfunction I commonly see is a result of nerve compression. The sensations of an orgasm travel to the brain along a nerve that exits the spine in the lumbar area of the back. Fully experienced, the nerve impulses create an electrifying sensation throughout a man's body, including an endorphin rush and a momentary high. The signals quickly travel from the penis to the brain and back, transmitting pleasure and the cues that lead to ejaculation. I wish I could more fully explain to women just how wonderful this sensation is. It's the reason that physically and emotionally healthy men desire passionately to recreate this feeling on a regular basis with their women! (Some men may even experience "goose bumps" as they ejaculate—the sympathetic nervous system's response to excitation.) But because this area is often misaligned or injured, the compression of the nerve inhibits the orgasm nerve impulses, resulting in less powerful orgasms and ejaculations. This is reason enough for every man to see a chiropractor trained in spinal manipulation!

PRE-EJACULATION DYSFUNCTION

I receive emails, phone calls for consultations and discussion with many women who have mates who ejaculate upon or right before penetration. My suggestion for anyone who ejaculates quickly would be to *slow down during the day*. This includes cutting back on adrenal gland stimulants: coffee, sugar and caffeine in general. The sympathetic nervous system is responsible for ejaculation. If it is over-stimulated, you may overreact to the moment and release prematurely.

DIABETES AND SEXUAL DYSFUNCTION

Diabetes is the third-highest killer of people in our country; I can even foresee it becoming number one as a result of our society's addiction to sugar, lack of exercise and obesity. The complications of diabetes can affect every tissue in the body. Patients who present a history of diabetes or even pre-diabetic tendencies are more apt to be pain sensitive, have higher rates of infection and generally seem to suffer from a large variety of health issues. Diabetes interferes with the movement and use of fuel (glucose) in the body, gradually decreasing pancreatic function. This increases insulin levels, which in turn creates inflammation in the body and reduced blood flow. Erections are built and maintained with blood flow in the genitals, so you can see how this disease plays a large role in erectile health.

Natural treatments for diabetes-related erectile dysfunction would include minimizing refined grain products that contain sugar. I always encourage my patients to exercise with weights, resistive bands, training equipment and aerobic activity. Losing weight is a step in the right direction because weight loss is critical for long-term blood sugar control. I routinely suggest that my patients request an HA1c (or hemoglobin A1c) test, which reveals the amount of glucose that has attached itself to the red blood cells over the last 120 days and is a good barometer to assess blood sugar issues.

PAIN SYNDROMES

I treat a variety of pain syndromes in my practice. Back and pelvic pain prevent many couples from having intercourse. Even if a couple is capable of intercourse, pain often limits the variety of sexual positions they can enjoy. Varying sexual positions keeps intimacy fresh and exciting, and a couple's relationship is bound to suffer when they don't have this wonderful variety available.

If you experience spinal pain during intercourse, schedule an assessment by a skilled chiropractor and also seek an experienced trainer to assist you in toning and strengthening your core muscles. Deb and I have worked out for years, and I'm absolutely certain that the strength we've gained as a result has enhanced our ability to engage in and enjoy intimate sexual contact.

I've had many patients come to my office complaining of pain radiating into the groin from their back. Three of these men were actually scheduled to have their left testicle medically removed as a solution to the problem—quite a drastic solution, if you ask me! All three men had misaligned pelvic bones. With appropriate assessment and spinal correction, their testicle pain went away. Each returned to their physician and was relieved to have avoided the surgery. If you are suffering from this pain syndrome, your pelvic alignment should be assessed by a health care provider who is skilled in natural spinal manipulation. Always rule out pathology, but seek a natural treatment first and foremost.

Pain may also be a culprit in places other than the reproductive organs. I recently had a consultation with a husband and wife; the husband was quite distraught because every time his wife had an orgasm she would develop a severe migraine. You can imagine that this was interfering with their sexual relationship! She completed a very detailed symptom survey form and I determined her pituitary gland was not up to full function. We supported the gland with a natural product and her migraines went away.

SUBLUXATION AND WHOLE-BODY HEALTH

I have extensive post-graduate training in spinal and whole-body structural bio-mechanics and I assess the function of the spine of every patient who comes into my office. Using x-rays and a physical examination, I search for any vertebral subluxation, meaning a misalignment of any of the 24 moveable spinal vertebrae, which then potentially compresses the nerves leaving the spinal cord as they connect to the organ and muscle tissues in the body. Your body communicates not only chemically or hormonally, as we have been discussing, but also via the nervous system, which, as I mentioned in the discussion on treating ED, can actually impair your sexual ability and function. Incorporating spinal correction or adjustments not only helps reduce your back and neck pain, but it also will improve your overall health! You would be wise to include the services of a skilled chiropractor as a part of your larger health and wellness plan.

A healthy spine is a healthy you. You will really enjoy the relief that comes with a spinal correction that minimizes any compression of nerves, as some chronic conditions like sinusitis, digestive distress, headaches and colon function can improve and be better managed by having your brain once again communicating with tissues via the nerves and spinal cord. Your nervous system sends 28 billion messages to be interpreted daily, from the brain cell to the tissue cell and then back again. You want this loop functioning optimally, as it allows your body to heal from the inside out, the way it was designed to do. On the other hand, the commonly accepted symptomatic or medical model of care, as so many of my new patients have reported to me that they have experienced with their previous health care providers, is to take a recommended medication or prescription for a trial or "wait and see" period that does not get to the root cause of the problem. While medications may manage the symptoms often initially caused or precipitated by the misalignment or subluxation stopping the brain-to-tissue-cell loop (think of it like your computer to your USB port to your printer), they do nothing to solve the real problem. The consistent completion of this loop is one of the reasons why my clients and patients respond to drugless care.

PEYRONIE'S DISEASE (AKA "BENT PENIS")

Another sexual challenge becoming more prevalent is Peyronie's disease. This condition results in painful, hardened, cord-like lesions (scar tissue known as "plaques") and abnormal curvature of the penis when erect. In addition, narrowing and/or shortening of the penis may occur. Pain felt in the early stages of the disease often resolves in 12 to 18 months. Erectile dysfunction, in varying degrees, often accompanies these symptoms in Peyronie's later stages. The condition may make sex painful and/or difficult, though many men report satisfactory intercourse in spite of the disease. Although it can affect men of any race and age, it's most commonly seen in Caucasian males above the age of 40. Peyronie's is not contagious, nor is it related in any way to cancer. The disease only affects men and is confined to the penis.

About 30 percent of men with Peyronie's disease develop fibrosis in other elastic tissues of the body, such as on the hand or foot, including Dupuytren's contracture of the hand (where the fingers bend towards the palm and cannot be straightened). An increased incidence in genetically related males suggests a genetic component. In my experience with patients, I've noticed two common causes: high copper found on tissue-hair mineral analysis resulting in adhesions, and low iodine found on the iodine loading test with lower than midline values seen on the T3 and T4 thyroid panel test. (See Chapter 15 for more insight on facilitating normal tissue function.)

If you're experiencing any of the symptoms of Peyronie's, you should see an experienced health care provider who has helped manage Peyronie's without surgery. I am commonly approached after I speak on hormonal challenges by men who have the same concern: "My doctor wants to operate on my penis. What should I do?" I usually suggest having a tissue-hair mineral analysis to determine copper and zinc ratios. High copper levels increase the risk of tissue-binding adhesions, as discussed above. Heightened zinc intake can bring copper to a more normal state. You should also avoid wheat, soy and sugar since they deplete zinc. The treatment protocol depends on the findings from your assessment. Also noteworthy is that Peyronie's is common after you have had a scope for kidney stones or an assessment where a urologist may have created distress to the pathway or urethra in your penis. Always ask if penetrating the penis for observation is necessary and inquire if there are other non-invasive procedures you could have instead.

CONDOM USE AND UNFULFILLED INTERCOURSE

This form of male sexual challenge is rarely discussed but has an extremely large impact on the sexual psyche of a man and the sexual health of a couple. The act of intercourse was designed for an incredibly intimate flesh-to-flesh encounter. One form of birth control inhibits this flesh-to-flesh encounter: the condom.

Let me share my own experience with you. My wife used birth control pills for the first six years of our marriage. Looking back,

I'm sure the pill altered her body chemistry, including her hormone balance, but we really didn't know any better back then and, to be honest, our sex life was great in every other regard. We decided to start a family and stopped using oral contraceptives. After our first son was born, Deb and I agreed that she would not go back on the birth control pill. For the next four years between her pregnancies we used condoms for contraception. Deb didn't mind this method, mainly because we threw the condom away and she didn't have to deal with my semen flowing out of her for the next couple of hours. My experience, however, was completely different.

Condom use over those four years had a drastic impact on our marriage, though it wasn't until years later that I was able to look back and recognize all that was occurring. After years of skin-to-skin intercourse with my wife, putting on a condom and losing that intimate contact took the spark out of our sex life for me. We were still having intercourse, but it was as though the intimacy of the act was gone. Men have an internal explosion of emotional sexual feelings with intimate skin-to-skin intercourse. I've attempted to explain this to Deb but it's almost like I don't have the words for it. A physical and arousing bonding called "sexual transmutation" occurs during this most intimate act that becomes even more intense as a man makes passionate love to a woman and then ejaculates inside her. Intercourse becomes much more than contact between sexual organs; the meeting of flesh actually fuses a couple together—mind, body and spirit. This is what the scriptures are speaking of when they talk about two becoming one flesh. A condom insulates partners from each other and from the skin-to-skin contact.

So, as I said, this constant lack of skin-to-skin intimacy with Deb had enormous repercussions. I suddenly felt disconnected from her sexually. Even though we continued to have sex, I felt like we weren't really being intimate. It drove me crazy, and it also drove me to drink! I drowned my pity party with alcohol, which only compounded our marital problems because I was nearly always high on "spirits." Of course, having sex with a drunk wasn't very appealing to Deb and soon she felt as sexually distant as I did.

I'm not saying that condoms were the reason I drank, but they were a major source of frustration for me. We had very limited sexual time together and drifted far apart. The alcohol temporarily distracted me from those frustrations but also decreased our sexual and emotional involvement. Deb was not pleased with me or the choices I was making, but she hung in there. I stopped drinking alcohol a few years after our youngest son was born. I know that if I had continued my excessive alcohol consumption, we more than likely would have divorced.

After our second son was born, I had a vasectomy. It was one of the wisest decisions we have ever made! It enables us to have very spontaneous sex without hesitation, and we don't have to stop and search for a condom or take the time to put one on. If you're currently using condoms, have a frank and honest discussion about the impact they are having on your sexual relationship. If either partner is suffering from a lack of skin-to-skin contact, discuss another method of birth control.

While we're talking about skin-to-skin contact, here's something for you to ponder: When a man ejaculates inside his woman, his seminal fluid is absorbed by her vaginal cells. Because it contains high levels of protein, semen is a source of cellular nutrition and a woman's body will absorb the protein in her man's ejaculate. In natural health care, using the proteins (the RNA and DNA) of one animal to treat another is called cell therapy or glandular therapy. After prolonged ejaculations (I'm talking about a number of years), a woman may actually start to take on some physical characteristics of her male partner. Look at the couples you know who have been married for a long time and you may notice they're beginning to resemble each other!

You may be struggling with one or more of the conditions addressed in this chapter, but be encouraged. You can have the mutually fulfilling sex life that you were designed to enjoy! Start by choosing one or two ways to naturally treat whatever is holding you back.

"MR. ED": MANAGING ERECTILE DYSFUNCTION – ACTIONS STEPS

☐ Journal what you eat and drink for one week. Do you recognize a pattern of sweets, grains and soda? If you do, schedule a family meeting and agree together to slowly incorporate healthy choices of organic vegetables and protein into your diet. Your well-being as well as your family's health will improve!

☐ Drink water from a pure source.

☐ Are you depressed, have high blood pressure or a history of heart disease? Find a proactive natural health care provider who can coach you from a prescription-based mindset to one that is a natural health-and-wellness way of life.

☐ If your EFAs are within normal, taking aspirin may do your body more harm than good. That baby aspirin may be causing your ED! Have an EFA blood spot test completed before deciding to add an aspirin a day to your health strategy.

☐ Walk a minimum of 20 minutes daily with your significant other or find another form of exercise that you can do together. If you drink alcohol and have erectile challenges, consider cutting back or quitting altogether.

☐ Be sure to read Chapters 13 and 15 on the adrenal glands and thyroid, respectively.

☐ Take advantage of nocturnal erections if you have ED difficulties during the day.

☐ Search for a contraceptive method that facilitates skin-to-skin contact.

NOTES

11

ARE YOU STIMULATING YOUR PARTNER?

If you're a typical man, the amount of sex you're actually having doesn't satisfy your sexual appetite. While libidos vary between individuals, men typically have higher sexual appetites than women. (This is more understandable when you consider that a sexual experience almost always results in climax for men, while the odds for women walking away sexually satisfied are much lower.) An unfortunate consequence of sexual frustration for men is that they often feel like any intimacy that occurs is at the whim of their partner. But the truth is that men have an incredible amount of control over the frequency of sexual intimacy within their relationship if they are willing to be considerate lovers who are concerned with their partner's needs as well as their own!

Would you like to have more sexually intimate times with your significant other? I'd like to suggest some things you can do that will guarantee her willingness—and even eagerness!—to have sex with you. The first is what you offer her with your own body. It's amazing to me how many men don't stop to consider their appearance. They have high standards for their woman (weight, makeup, clothing, etc.) but take very little time to consider what they are bringing to the bedroom. I have one patient who confided in me that her husband constantly picks and eats the scabs off his skin. Are you surprised that it makes her cringe to think of being intimate with him? I'm not! So let's take an honest look at something men far too often overlook: personal hygiene.

PERSONAL HYGIENE

Do you get a haircut regularly? Trim nose and ear hair? Keep your nails clean and trimmed? I know a woman whose husband is a contractor. He's a hard worker and it shows on his hands. She told me that it was actually painful for her when he ran his hands over her body because they were so torn up. Instead of reacting in frustration every time he scraped his hands across her skin, this woman prayed for wisdom in responding to her husband. The insight that came was for her to tenderly care for her husband's hands. Now she occasionally washes his hands, exfoliates them with a natural scrub and rubs lotion into them. Not only does it solve the problem, but it's become an occasional part of their foreplay. Her husband enjoys the tender attention and this wonderful wife receives a spiritual blessing. She could choose to complain and turn down her husband's advances, leading to his resentment and frustration. Instead, she blesses her husband and, in turn, their marriage.

Do you shave regularly? Whiskers can actually burn a woman's sensitive skin, especially if you have gray facial hair, which is extremely coarse. Facial hair means less area to shave, but you should consider what impact it might be having on your sex life. In fact, have you ever thought to ask your partner if she even likes your mustache and/or beard? If I knew that my wife would be more attracted to me and want more sex if I had a handlebar mustache, you can bet I'd start growing one today! But if facial hair bothers her, shave regularly. The benefits are worth a few more minutes in front of the mirror.

A large part of personal hygiene is your body odor. Your body could radiate a pungent fragrance; it should be a pleasant one! Do you shower daily? Women have a very keen sense of smell; they are much more sensitive than men. I can't think of anything less appealing than having a sweaty, smelly naked spouse trying to wrap themselves around me. Before you approach your significant other, make sure you have showered and put on deodorant and clean clothes.

Speaking of body aroma, women are very concerned about their own personal hygiene, specifically their vaginal scent. Vaginas are not fragrance free. Hormonal changes and the woman's level of physical activity all contribute to the way a vagina radiates its own fragrance. If your woman feels embarrassed by her scent, find ways to help her carve out time for a shower or bath. Put the kids to bed while she freshens up. She will be thankful for your help and it will give her time to relax and get in the mood. If it's possible, join her in the shower and offer to scrub her back. (The shower is a great place for occasional "On, In and Out" sex if you don't have much time, and it allows her to quickly wash up afterward.)

Do your feet reek? Mine used to when I consumed alcohol and my liver and kidney function was compromised. How is your breath? Chronic bad breath can be a sign of poor digestion. Stop drinking fluids with your meals, as too much liquid will dilute the enzymes in your stomach and interfere with digestion. As that food sits putrefying in your stomach, it releases gases that can lead to bad breath. Talk to your natural health care provider for advice on a drugless digestive aid. And, by the way, I would not use sugar or sugar substitute–based breath fresheners. They will compromise your adrenal gland function, which we will discuss in Chapter 13.

Do you smoke or chew tobacco? If you do, you're asking your woman to kiss a chimney! You can imagine the damper that puts on her desire to be intimate with you.

And while we're talking about smells, it may be time to update your cologne. Do you still have the same old bottle from five years ago? It's probably stale by now. Set up a date with your significant other and go shopping together for a new scent. You'd spend money on a game of golf, fishing tackle or any other hobby you may have; why not invest in your sex life? Cologne is an easy way to help put your lady in the mood or at least help her start thinking about it. You should purchase one ounce spray bottles because the oil on your skin as well as contaminants on your fingers can alter the scent of cologne that must be applied by hand. Go to a men's store, a large department store or a specialty store where the products are fresh and purchase a new fragrance.

Is your wardrobe clean, neat and well put together? You don't have to turn into a *GQ* model, and that's probably not even what your woman wants. But I can guarantee that she will appreciate a well-dressed man and be more open to sex if you approach her clean and looking great!

Even more important than wooing your woman physically is meeting her emotional desires. Men who are focused on their own needs while ignoring their partner's are understandably going to get turned down again and again. But when you consider her and make her requests your priority, she will be more likely to respond sexually.

TAKING TIME TO CONNECT

Are you listening to your woman? Putting down the paper, turning off the TV, turning away from the computer and really listening? If you aren't, don't expect her to listen to your pleas for intimacy; she is feeling ignored and unloved. In the morning, ask about her plans for the day. In the evening, remember those plans and ask how they went. Trust me, she will immediately recognize and appreciate that you remembered what she had going on during the day! Talk about more than "business as usual" subjects: the kids, the house, the calendar, her job. What are her dreams? Let her know you are interested in every aspect of her life.

Another important need you should be meeting for your significant other is quality time together. She wants more than your paycheck and an occasional romp in the bedroom—she wants you! That means carving out time for just the two of you; you should be doing it, so write it down in your calendar! You will undoubtedly be hoping that a date night will include sex, but don't pressure her in that regard. Just enjoy spending time together. If it leads to sex, great; if it doesn't, you've still made an investment in your relationship that will pay off in the future.

One of the easiest ways to bless your partner is to simply help her. Do you help her clear the dishes from the table after meals? Do you carry heavy loads of laundry up the stairs for her? Does she put the kids to bed alone every night? She shouldn't! Help her get them ready or, better yet, take over a few nights a week and give her a chance to relax. Put your dirty laundry in the hamper instead of leaving it on the floor where you take it off. Those things sound simple, but trust me—they go a long way!

Gentlemen, the only thing necessary for you to want to have sex is the smallest piece of visual stimulus and a functioning reproductive system. Your female partner was made differently, and before you resent her, take a step back for one moment and appreciate that she is functioning just the way nature intended. She needs relationship in order to desire sex with you. This is a great blessing to your partnership because it forces you to stay connected with her in order to get your sexual needs met. If she didn't have that need for relationship, the two of you might very well drift apart without even realizing what's happening. Instead of feeling offended that you seem to have to pay a price for sex with your woman (in the form of errands, backrubs, daily showers, etc.), be thankful that she has built in her a deep need for connection that forces you both to come together.

VARIETY IS THE SPICE OF LIFE

Would you eat the same lunch every day for the rest of your life? Of course not—how boring! Your sex life should be the same way. Variety is the spice of life and your sex life should be just as exciting. Instead of viewing sex as a means to the goal of ejaculation, slow down and enjoy exploring each other's bodies. Make the journey as wonderful as the destination.

What you actually do in the bedroom is totally dependent on what you decide together as a couple. Don't pressure your partner into sexual behavior that makes her feel uncomfortable. Discuss what you desire and mutually agree on your time together.

You have an amazing amount of control over your sex life. Ask your wife or significant other to tell you how you can serve her better and meet her needs. You'll probably be blessed with a lot more sex, but the payoff is even greater than that: You'll be working as partners to increase your love for each other.

ARE YOU STIMULATING YOUR PARTNER? – ACTION STEPS

- ☐ What changes do you need to make in your personal hygiene to become more attractive to your woman?

- ☐ How can you become a better listener?

- ☐ What do you need to do to have more quality time with your wife or significant other? Stop right now and schedule a date night with her.

☐ In what little ways can you help around the house? Choose one or two and start doing them today. And don't announce them to your woman like you are expecting a sexual payback! Just quietly start serving her and trust that there will be a reward.

12

IT'S MORE THAN "ON, IN AND OUT"

The longer I'm married, the more I realize how differently my wife and I are wired. I have a high libido and am relentless in my pursuit of her. She enjoys our sexual encounters but is not always as passionate about having sex; she's much more fervent about spending time together and sharing what's going on in our lives. Our experience with couples has proven this trend; women are much more concerned with the relational and romantic aspects of their marriage. In contrast, candid conversations with married men generally come to a vastly different conclusion: Men's priorities are sex, food and recreation. Unfortunately, we've come to realize that most men are either in denial or ignorant to the fact that men and women differ physically and emotionally in their approach to sexuality.

In my practice, women commonly express their frustration that they feel sexually rushed by their partners, who move too quickly in their intimate time. Women need time to warm up, conversation, touching, caressing and foreplay, and too many of them walk away from sex unfulfilled because those requirements for orgasm are unmet. The media promotes this lopsided sexual experience with passionate—and completely unrealistic—love scenes full of fireworks, earthquakes and orgasms, all in the span of a few minutes! We've coined a phrase for this kind of sexual encounter: "On, In and Out!" Many women feel exactly this way: Their lover wants to get on them, get in them and then get out and back to the next task. It's almost impossible for a woman to walk away from this kind of "lovemaking" with any satisfaction or the desire for more.

There are exceptions to this rule, and there are even couples where the female is more interested in sex, but I have found the "On, In and Out" experience to be surprisingly common. So why do healthy men seem to always want to have sex? Well, it's possible for both men and women to desire sex, but only men *need* to have sex. This is a crucial difference between men and women, a fact very few people even recognize. But once you understand the physiological drives that make men pursue sex, it becomes a great blessing in the bedroom.

WHY MEN NEED SEX

In every man's body there are two small glands called the "seminal vesicles." These glands have a profound effect on men's sexual desire and behavior, though most men aren't even aware of their existence or function. I learned about them while taking an anatomy class and actually dissected them in a cadaver. The seminal vesicles are probably the most neglected tissue discussed in human sexuality.

Each seminal vesicle looks like an overcooked, deflated hot dog. They're about four or five inches long, and nestled inside each vesicle is a coiled tube that continuously creates seminal fluid. Since they never cease production, the seminal vesicles keep filling up after each ejaculation. As they fill with seminal fluid, the vesicles swell and stretch out much like a coiled garden hose tends to stretch out when filled with water. The seminal vesicles can't release any of the seminal fluid other than by ejaculation, and when ejaculation doesn't occur for a prolonged period of time, the swelling of the vesicles can actually make a man's testicles ache. This may seem unusual to women, especially because it sounds like an odd and ridiculous excuse to get them into bed, but it's true!

When the seminal vesicles are full of fluid, we men have a few options to release the pressure. The most obvious is to initiate sex with our partner. If that doesn't happen, we may fantasize about other women while engaging in self-stimulation (masturbation). We may even experience ejaculation as a result of a sexual dream, fondly called a "wet dream." It's also not uncommon to discover leakage of the seminal fluid in our underwear if the pressure isn't relieved by ejaculation.

This normal sexual process involves much more than genitals, however; it's closely connected to your largest sexual organ: your brain! Closely surrounding the seminal vesicle is a network of pressure-sensitive nerves called the "vesicle plexus." A plexus is a group of tightly knit nerves with a specific function, and this particular group of nerves alerts the hypothalamus of the amount of pressure being placed on it by the swelling of the seminal vesicles via the information superhighway of the spinal cord. The hypothalamus, in turn, contains a unique structure of specialized "neural circuits," which are specifically designed to trigger sexual arousal in response to the messages received from the vesicle plexus. So as each seminal vesicle swells and presses against the vesicle plexus, a message is sent to the hypothalamus that essentially says, "Too much pressure! Think about having some sex up there!"

The hypothalamus faithfully responds by stimulating the release of testosterone (by the testes and adrenal glands) into the bloodstream. Testosterone is the sex hormone at work in both men and women's bodies that triggers a conscious awareness of sexual need.

A word on testosterone is in order. In my clinical practice, I've observed an epidemic of men who are unable to respond to the thought of sexual intimacy because they are simply overworked, stressed and eating too many toxic foods. In short, your endocrine system is exhausted! This is easily treated with a glandular tissue supplement and minerals to revitalize this essential part of the brain; in my practice, we use a product with an ingredient called maca root. If you have no desire for sex, it's not necessarily psychological; it may simply be that your body is overloaded and unable to function properly. There are other reasons for a diminished libido, which were discussed in Chapter 10 on erectile dysfunction, but a low-functioning hypothalamus is one that is often overlooked.

So if a man has recently ejaculated and his seminal vesicles are relatively empty, no pressure is placed on the vesicle plexus and no message is sent to the hypothalamus. No message means no dump of testosterone into the bloodstream. No testosterone dump, then no extreme awareness of sexual desire. However, if ejaculation hasn't occurred in a while and the vesicles are filled to bursting with fluid, vesicle plexus sends a message, the hypothalamus dumps out testosterone and your average male turns into a panting, sexual beast! The knowledge of this wonderful system should bring a sigh of relief to both men and women. Your woman now won't think you are a sex-crazed maniac, but just operating the way you were intended. The process explains why a man who recently had sex can go about his business focused and determined, while a man who has a large buildup of seminal fluid can't walk by a lingerie store without an intense hormonal arousal.

IT'S ALL ABOUT TIMING

The timing is unique for each man; some may go days before sufficient seminal buildup starts the process, while others may go only hours. But once the proverbial dam breaks, a man's mind is sensitized to every sexual stimulus he comes across. Involuntarily, a man finds himself intensely and powerfully attracted by sexual thoughts and fantasies, including acute awareness of the women in his immediate vicinity. As a result of this purely biological function, men are subject throughout their adult lives to the compellingly distractive and recurrent sexual cycle of involuntary arousal, bodily excitation and ejaculation followed by temporary serenity.

This is by no means an excuse for immorality or callous treatment of women. I always tell my female readers and patients that if their husband or boyfriend ever tries to use this biological system as justification for brutish and selfish demands, they have my full permission to get out this book and hit him with it! But this knowledge does give women the wonderful opportunity to understand your sexual needs and drives and to help you cope with distracting sexual impulses by offering a warm and welcoming sexual outlet in your relationship bed.

This isn't to say there's not a place for "On, In and Out" sex within a relationship. There are occasions in our routine when Deb is not so interested in sex but she recognizes that I have a dire need for release. Because we're honest and open in our communication, I can express that need to her without fear that she'll roll her eyes and label me a "sex maniac." And because she realizes that not every sexual encounter has to include fireworks and earthquake orgasms, she willingly and lovingly allows me an "On, In and Out" experience (sometimes called a "quickie"). She also knows that I am much easier to get along with when I've had that sexual release.

I have daily, and I do mean daily, conversations with men who I know are frustrated with their sex lives and the lack of vaginal intercourse. I recently had one man who was angry tell me that he connects with his wife one time a year on his birthday! I suggested the "quick" moment together and he rolled his eyes, telling me that it was just not going to happen. I told him that he and his wife need to sit down and talk! He is ready to throw in the towel and get a divorce. I truly believe that if couples connected sexually more often, there would be much less divorce. You may have to show your partner this chapter to start your conversation.

A word of advice here: Your woman will be much more willing to engage in healthy "On, In and Out" sex if she knows that in the near future you will take the time to have a prolonged sexual encounter with her that includes tender caresses, loving conversation, lots of foreplay and a focus on her sexual fulfillment. If all of your sex is the down-and-out, over-in-three-minutes kind, expect her to grow more and more resentful and less and less willing to consider your swelling seminal vesicles over time!

Timing is incredibly important when it comes to the two of you coming together in a mutually satisfying sexual rendezvous. And women aren't exempt from timing, as you know if you've ever dealt with a partner suffering from premenstrual syndrome![1] Shortly after finishing menstruation, a woman's hormone level peaks. This is in preparation for ovulation, when a woman is at her most fertile for 24-48 hours. It makes sense, then, that women are designed to be more sexually aware at this time in their cycle. You would be wise to become very informed about your partner's menstrual cycles, because it will greatly benefit you in the bedroom! A few days after her period ends is the time to initiate long, intimate love-making sessions; it's when she's most physically and emotionally responsive and most likely to achieve an orgasm. Following ovulation (which generally occurs about 14 days after her period starts), the sex hormones decline in preparation for menstruation if there's no fertilization and pregnancy. These few weeks after ovulation are generally marked by declining sexual interest, and it's when she will probably be relieved if you understand that she's not so willing to jump through sexual hoops. She may be experiencing the preparation for menstruation with its mood swings, bloating, etc., which understandably doesn't make her feel very sexually appealing or adventurous. This is the time for gently requesting "On,

In and Out" intimacy. You might approach her by saying, "I know you're not feeling very sexual right now, but I would love to just be with you and enjoy some sexual release. I want to direct my desires toward you and not feel so overwhelmed by other stimuli. Would you consider meeting that need for me?" If you have another way of saying this, then by all means. Trust me, your woman will be astounded by your gentleness and consideration as well as touched by your vulnerability.

DON'T FORGET TO DATE YOUR LOVER

Now that you realize how important timing is for a mutually fulfilling sexual experience, it makes sense to put some thought into when you should have sex. Plan to have sex?! Absolutely! Although occasionally sex will occur spontaneously, the demands of work, family and friends prevent those thrilling surprises from happening very often. A smart couple will intentionally carve out time to spend together, which may or may not include sex. For example, when I'm on the road for a few days, I often purchase flowers or a small gift for Deb. If Deb is out of town, I'll welcome her home with romantic music playing, candles in our bedroom and possibly even some homemade whipped cream. Deb does the same for me, occasionally purchasing lingerie and preparing in ways she knows will really turn me on. What a wonderful way to reconnect after an absence!

It actually seems crazy not to plan for sex. I see business travelers at airports who are totally drained and patients at my practice who are worn out. I see couples who work shifts and barely see each other or who work multiple jobs to make ends meet. If they aren't planning for intimate time together, I can almost guarantee it isn't happening. The plans don't always have to include sex, either, although time spent focusing on each other usually leads to physical intimacy. Even if it doesn't, your relationship will be strengthened and the loving feelings that are developed will certainly increase the odds for sex in the future. All of this planning is really nothing more than dating your mate. Don't let being married or in a committed relationship stop you from dating each other! Your plans can be as simple as a walk, a bike ride or a picnic.

I'll never forget a date I had with Deb while traveling in Florida. I had done my planning—I took massage oil, candles and an MP3 player with her favorite music. We had very intense whole-body sex without the stress of work and children. When we're attending business seminars, we take time to have spontaneous sex in the hotel room. These planned times of intimacy have truly been one of our secret weapons as a couple and have kept our marriage amazingly passionate. They'll do the same for you!

YOUR MIND GOES WHERE YOUR ENERGY FLOWS

Now that you realize how incredibly different men and women are sexually, let me offer some specific suggestions that will greatly improve your sex life. An important concept to remember is that where your mind goes your energy flows. Simply put, if you desire more sex, you should be devoting energy in the pursuit of that goal! Sometimes I talk with men who are experiencing relationship challenges, yet they're so busy scheduling a golf game or a hunting trip that it's almost inevitable they aren't having any sex with their woman. Many men don't consider romancing their significant other or creating the emotional and physical intimacy that will almost guarantee them a sexual interlude. You may still get her in bed with this kind of thinking, but to have an absolutely wonderful sex life you need to include her in your day-planner and consider the times that she might want to be intimate, not just the times you want sex. This may be the most important relationship lesson you can learn; your mate, believe it or not, desires and wants your companionship, love, support and time. When those needs are met, she will almost assuredly also want sex!

First, devote time to quality conversation and romantic moments together. Happy relationships are based on deep friendship. Isn't it uncomfortable when you're with a couple who obviously aren't friends, but enemies? When friends become unfriendly, we walk away from the friendship, yet too many spouses treat each other terribly and then wonder why their relationship suffers. If you wouldn't make sarcastic remarks to a friend, you certainly shouldn't be making them to your wife or girlfriend. If you wouldn't put down a friend in front of a crowd, you shouldn't do it to your significant other, either. In fact, building her up in front of other people makes a huge statement to your woman—and the crowd—about how much you value her. The words you speak will build your house or tear it down, so consider them carefully. For the same reason, don't hang around people who consistently speak negatively about their spouses. Sometimes when a group of all men or all women gets together, they spend much of their time putting down the opposite sex. This only leads to dissatisfaction! Be the brave person who redirects the conversation toward something edifying about your mate; it will bring gentle conviction to the others and they'll admire you for it. It will also bless your mate when she hears that you've been talking about her (saying good things!) behind her back.

CREATING PASSION

Start to become a pursuer of your woman instead of just a pursuer of sex. This means that meeting her sexual needs should become as important to you as meeting your sexual needs. This comes naturally for many men who get enormous emotional satisfaction from stimulating their wives or girlfriends and sharing their climax. Other men haven't yet realized that half of the pleasure of sex is enjoying your partner's orgasm as much as your own! Sadly, many women have never achieved orgasm, and it's somewhat stunning that they still desire intimacy at all. Gentlemen—trust me!—it's in your best interest to put a smile on her face. If you're unsure about what she needs, bring it up in a quiet moment and let her know that you are willing to learn. This could mean swallowing your pride, but the payoff in intimacy will be worth it. Remember that what she tells you may include what not to do as much as what she does enjoy. Don't pressure her to perform, but reassure her that this is something you're willing to work on when she's in the mood. Take your time and enjoy learning how to be a considerate lover.

And while we're talking about meeting her needs, it would be in your best interest to start doing those extra little chores around the house that would take stress off of her. Until her "To Do List" is finished in the evening, sex is just another chore! Ask her what you can do to help. As suggested earlier, offer to put the children to bed so she has time for a bath. When men tell me they're dissatisfied with their sex lives, I ask a few questions right off the bat: Do you empty the dishwasher? Pick up after yourself? Lower the toilet seat? Squeeze the toothpaste at the end? Help with dinner? Don't be resentful, feeling like you are "paying" for sex by being helpful in this way. No, you are investing in a relationship that gives huge dividends when properly cared for!

BE A MODEL OF LOVE AND PASSION

Perhaps you are in a difficult position, desiring changes in your sex life when your mate doesn't seem to care. Please be encouraged! We've seen one person start making changes in their health and their approach to sex, and the disinterested partner slowly wakes up as they see positive results. Couples like this often become partners in improving their relationship. Determine that you will make healthy and positive choices despite what your mate does or doesn't do.

I just received an email from a woman who subscribes to my weekly e-tips and is familiar with the work I'm doing on the subject of sex and romance. She was excited to inform me that she had recently been communicating with her husband about what he could do to please her sexually. Her husband often rushed through sex and she had never expressed wanting anything different. After a few honest discussions, he became an expert at pleasing her and they are enjoying the best sex of their 35-year marriage! Every couple can improve upon the wonderful blessing of sexuality. It's my hope that your relationship bed will be filled with honesty, tenderness and joy!

IT'S MORE THAN "ON, IN AND OUT" – ACTION STEPS

☐ Reserve some quiet time to candidly discuss your libidos. Whose is higher/lower? How do you feel about the frequency of your lovemaking? Do you need to make adjustments to satisfy the needs of your partner?

☐ How often is your lovemaking slow and tender, and how often is it the "On, In and Out" kind? How do you feel about these percentages? (Remember that "On, In and Out" sex has a place in your relationship as long as you both feel satisfied by its frequency.)

☐ What changes can be made to ensure mutually satisfying intimacy as often as each partner desires it, and "On, In and Out" sex as often as each partner is agreeable?

☐ Are you willing to humbly listen to your mate's requests and help her in this capacity?

☐ What are some common reasons that you turn down sex? Are there things your partner can do to make you more willing to have sex?

☐ Are you intentionally planning times for intimacy, whether or not they include lovemaking?

13

YOUR ADRENAL GLANDS: THE MOST IMPORTANT BODY PART YOU'VE NEVER HEARD OF

The conventional medical model is very compartmentalized, breaking the human body down into individual systems. While this concept is useful for instructional purposes, in reality, our systems don't function independently of each other. Your body is a complex, interdependent network of systems whose functions impact one another in profound ways. Unfortunately, Western medicine has generally treated hormonal dysfunction with medication and ignored the delicate balance of all of the components involved in hormonal health. One key player in that system is the adrenal glands, which have a role in male hormonal function including a suppressed libido in men and vaginal dryness in women.

I encourage you to read this chapter slowly in order to fully grasp all the truths it contains. Each new piece of information adds to the foundation of personal health and optimal (rarely correlated) hormonal function, including blood sugar, blood pressure, pain syndromes, which translate to things like energy, heart function and back pain.

As mentioned in Chapter 1, the adrenal glands are located atop each kidney and are about the size of a walnut. As an important member of the endocrine system, these glands work closely with the pituitary, pancreas and thyroid. One of their many functions is to help the body cope with stress. For our purposes in this chapter, we'll focus on the role these potent glands play in your hormonal health and function.

PHYSIOLOGY OF THE ADRENAL GLANDS

The adrenal glands are comprised of a large outer portion called the cortex and a smaller inner portion called the medulla. The cortex and medulla have different but very significant roles in hormonal function. The medulla secretes epinephrine and norepinephrine, two hormones responsible for the body's "fight-or-flight" response to stress. The cortex produces over 50 different types of hormones in three major classes:

- glucocorticoids
- mineralocorticoids
- androgens

The most important glucocorticoid is cortisol. When cortisol production is too low, the body's ability to deal with stress is markedly reduced. We will discuss the important role of cortisol in further detail later in this chapter. Mineralocorticoids such as aldosterone (a hormone that causes the tubules of the kidneys to retain sodium and water) modulate the delicate balance of minerals in the cells, especially sodium and potassium, and play a part in blood pressure regulation. Stress increases the release of aldosterone, causing sodium retention. The result is water retention and high blood pressure. When high blood pressure is treated with prescription medication, which is the norm in our society, a common side effect for men is erectile dysfunction. The stress-induced release of aldosterone also results in a loss of potassium and magnesium, which wreaks havoc on your body. Magnesium is involved in many enzymatic reactions throughout multiple systems; low magnesium plays a role in a variety of serious conditions in men, including cardiac arrhythmias, blood sugar stress, muscle cramping and constipation.

The adrenal cortex produces sex hormones in small but potent amounts. (See figure below.) An exception is DHEA, a weak androgenic hormone. DHEA, together with testosterone and estrogen, are made from pregnenolone, which in turn comes from cholesterol. Pregnenolone also leads to the production of progesterone and is one of the transition steps in the production of cortisol. Pregnenolone is therefore one of the significant intermediate hormones being produced in the hormonal cascade. Prolonged deficiencies in pregnenolone will lead to reduction of both glucocorticoids (cortisol) and mineralocorticoids (aldosterone).

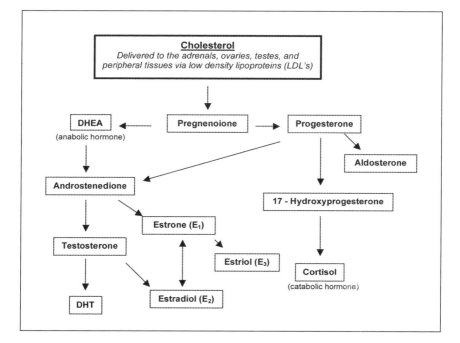

Cortisol is a very significant hormone, protecting the body from excessive daily pressure by:

Normalizing blood sugar: Cortisol increases blood sugar levels in the body, providing the energy necessary for the fight-or-flight response to danger. Cortisol works in tandem with insulin from the pancreas to provide adequate glucose to the cells for energy. More stress requires more energy, which explains why you crave refined carbohydrates and sweets when you are stressed. In adrenal fatigue, more cortisol is secreted during the early stages of stress until eventually the adrenal glands become exhausted and cortisol output is reduced. Blood sugar balance is disrupted, cholesterol is likely to increase and you may experience more pain throughout your body. All of this occurs because your body is caught in the vicious and demanding cycle of producing pregnenolone, which in turn increases cortisol and keeps your body in a state of constant agitation.

Anti-inflammatory response: Cortisol is a powerful anti-inflammatory agent. When you experience a minor injury or a muscle strain, your body's inflammatory cascade is initiated, leading to swelling and redness (commonly seen when an ankle is sprained or from an insect bite). Cortisol is secreted as a part of the anti-inflammatory response to control the response from the white blood cell "warriors" from the immune system. Its objective is to remove and prevent swelling and redness of nearly all tissues. These anti-inflammatory responses prevent mosquito bites from enlarging, eyes from swelling due to allergies, etc.

Immune system suppression: People with high levels of cortisol (which, as just discussed, has been released by the adrenals in a response to protect the body from a compensatory overreaction by the body) will eventually also have a suppressed immune system—the reason why you may get "sick" while under stress. What happens is the cortisol influences cells that participate in the immune reaction, especially white blood cells. Cortisol suppresses white blood cells and other "fighter cells" whose purpose is to protect the body from threats such as bacteria, fungus, viruses and cancer. Lowered immunity results in increased sickness and disease.

The Story of Stress in Your Body

People with adrenal fatigue cannot tolerate stress and are likely to succumb to severe nervous tension. As their stress increases, progressively higher levels of cortisol are required. When the cortisol level cannot rise in response to the situation at hand (job stress, hectic schedules, financial concerns, chronic marital or family challenges), it is impossible to maintain a body that is fully prepared to react appropriately to stress.

Cortisol sustains life through opposite but related regulatory actions: releasing and activating the body's defense mechanisms and shutting down and modifying those same mechanisms to prevent damage or cell loss.

The adrenal glands are directed via the hypothalamus-pituitary-adrenal (HPA) loop or axis, as discussed in Chapter 6 on weight loss. There is an existing negative feedback loop that governs the amount of adrenal hormones secreted under normal circumstances. For example, the HPA axis adjusts cortisol levels according to the body's need via a hormone called adrenocorticotrophic hormone (ACTH), which is secreted by the pituitary gland in response to signals from the hypothalamus, your body's CEO. This is a part of the weight loss loop.

When the ACTH attaches to the walls of the adrenal glands, a chain reaction occurs within the cell. This leads to the release of cholesterol, which is manufactured into pregnenolone, the first hormone in adrenal metabolism (See figure on page 187). Subsequently, cortisol is released into the bloodstream and moves throughout the body and back to the hypothalamus, where it is measured. This completes the negative feedback loop. In the human hormonal system, the negative feedback loop is designed to limit the production of each hormone.

This whole process is an amazing part of your physiology. When cared for, your body is kept in a constant state of homeostasis, or balance. Unfortunately, many people exist in a constant state of prolonged stress, and the increased cortisol levels that result blunt the negative feedback response. The delicate balance between the sympathetic and parasympathetic nervous systems is threatened as the sympathetic revs up to address the impending danger that increased cortisol levels have announced. As the parasympathetic system is pushed aside, so are many of its sexual functions, including vaginal lubrication in women and, as you've learned, the ability to produce and maintain an erection in men.

A body that is constantly flooded with the stress hormone cortisol is a body in distress. Why the constant stress? There are multiple reasons. A diet full of sugary foods creates a challenge for the adrenal glands. A stressful job, family problems, a fast-paced life—all lead to inflammation, which leads to increased cholesterol, which, when called on, jump-starts the production of cortisol. Taking cholesterol-lowering medications can reduce cholesterol and thus cortisol, but it often leads to erectile dysfunction. One problem is "solved" and a new one is created.[1]

Stress, then, induces the following responses in your body:

- Reduced insulin sensitivity, reduced glucose (or blood sugar) utilization and increased blood sugar lead to diabetes and the potential for erectile dysfunction if the disease is not properly managed.

- Reduced natural white blood "killer" cells in the body lead to infections such as herpes, yeast overgrowth, bacterial and viral infections. Women may experience chronic vaginal yeast infestation and men may develop genital rash and fungus on the toes or athlete's foot.

■ An increased loss in bone mass (as calcium absorption is blocked and demineralization of bone occurs) results in bone structures. I have seen this in men's low backs, shoulders, necks and generalized osteoporosis in those who have played contact sports, worked in construction with heavy lifting and/or have a history of active duty in the military.

■ Increased fat accumulation around the waist and protein breakdown lead to loss of muscle tone and the inability to lose weight.

■ Increased water and salt retention lead to high blood pressure.[2]

■ Estrogen saturation and/or dominance in men can lead to feminization, increased breast size, skinny arms and legs, prostate challenges and cancer, and even breast cancer.

Now you know what a hormonal reaction to stress looks like on paper, but what does it look like in real life? Imagine you're at work and your boss raises his voice to you. Here's what happens in your body from a hormonal perspective as the stress response kicks in:

1. Your hypothalamus signals your pituitary gland to release adrenocorticotrophic hormone (ACTH).

2. The ACTH stimulates the adrenal medulla to secrete epinephrine and the adrenal cortex to secrete cortisol and other hormones.

3. The epinephrine increases your heart rate.

4. The cortisol causes increased sweat production.

5. Both cortisol and epinephrine increase muscle tension. Digestion slows as blood is diverted away from organs that are less important to the fight-or-flight response.

6. The sympathetic nervous system is on high alert, dominating the parasympathetic nervous system. In an

agitated state, your body is more concerned with survival
than with ancillary functions (such as being intimate with
your mate) that are less essential in a state of emergency.

You arrive home after a tough day, and just when sexual intimacy
might be a wonderful release of tension and stress, which would
improve your situation, the last thing your body wants to do or is
capable of doing is performing the sexual act!

MEN, ADRENAL HEALTH AND SEX

Women have a larger network of hormones requiring harmony
than you do, but you can just as easily experience adrenal fatigue.
Men commonly work at high-stress jobs, consume diets lacking in
good nutrition and may live life more recklessly than our female
counterparts. All of these factors challenge the hormonal system;
the result is dominance by the sympathetic nervous system.

As you age and experience chronic stress, your body becomes less
effective at producing the necessary steroids for sexual function. If
your belly is 40 inches or more and your legs and arms are starting
to look like toothpicks, your androgens are not at a sufficient level
to promote muscle strength and integrity. This is a very common
and serious condition prevalent in our culture. As I've described,
men who are 45 think they're 19, and yet they have the hormonal
capacity of a 55-year-old. And you wonder why you need to take a
pill to get an erection!

THE ADRENAL GLAND ASSESSMENT

Do you experience:

- ☐ difficulty getting up in the morning?
- ☐ continuing fatigue that is not relieved by sleep and rest?
- ☐ lethargy, lack of energy to perform normal daily activities?
- ☐ sugar cravings?
- ☐ salt cravings?
- ☐ allergies?
- ☐ digestion problems?
- ☐ increased effort needed for everyday tasks?
- ☐ decreased interest in sex?
- ☐ decreased ability to handle stress?
- ☐ increased time needed to recover from illness, injury or traumas?
- ☐ lightheadedness or dizziness when standing up quickly?
- ☐ low mood?
- ☐ less enjoyment or happiness with life?
- ☐ symptoms that worsen if meals are skipped or inadequate?
- ☐ your thoughts being less focused—brain fog?
- ☐ poor memory?
- ☐ decreased tolerance for stress, noise, disorder?
- ☐ not really feeling awake until after 10 a.m.?
- ☐ an afternoon slump between 3 p.m. and 4 p.m.?
- ☐ feeling better after supper?
- ☐ getting a "second wind" in the evening and staying up late?
- ☐ decreased productivity?
- ☐ the feeling that you have to keep moving—that if you stop, you get tired?
- ☐ feeling overwhelmed by all that needs to be done?
- ☐ feeling that it takes all of your energy to do what you have to do—that there's nothing left over for anything or anyone else?

FACTORS LEADING TO ADRENAL FATIGUE

Which of the following are a part of your current life experience?

- ☐ White sugar and white flour products
- ☐ Stimulants
- ☐ Lack of relaxation
- ☐ Negative thinking
- ☐ Smoking
- ☐ Energy drinks
- ☐ Antacids
- ☐ Non-prescription drug use
- ☐ Devitalized food
- ☐ Psychological stress
- ☐ Unfulfilling employment
- ☐ Persistent fears
- ☐ Unfulfilling relationships
- ☐ Emotional stress
- ☐ Surgery
- ☐ Lack of sleep
- ☐ Unhealthy diet filled with junk food
- ☐ Inability to address your feelings/denial
- ☐ Consuming trans fats and/or rancid fats
- ☐ Infection, acute or chronic
- ☐ Financial stress
- ☐ Persistent negative stressors
- ☐ Sedentary lifestyle
- ☐ Fun or enjoyment deprivation
- ☐ Excessive exercise
- ☐ Allergies
- ☐ Death of a loved one
- ☐ Caffeine
- ☐ Alcoholism
- ☐ Prescription drug use
- ☐ Toxins
- ☐ Relationship/marital stress
- ☐ Hormonal imbalances
- ☐ Repeated traumas
- ☐ Conventional hormone replacement therapy
- ☐ Workaholism

I suggest looking over these two assessments to see how many symptoms and factors you recognize in your own life. If you're experiencing sexual challenges and your overall personal health is not up to par, you should commit to making some changes. It will require discipline and new habit patterns. Many of the changes are actually counter-cultural in our fast-paced world, but your physical and sexual health is worth the effort! Start slowly by choosing a few new habits. As you are successful and your health starts to improve, it will give you great satisfaction and the motivation to do even more for your body and your sex life.

THE SYMPATHETIC AND PARASYMPATHETIC NERVOUS SYSTEMS

We've touched on the two significant players for favorable hormonal health—the sympathetic and parasympathetic nervous systems. It will be helpful for you to know if your body is sympathetic or parasympathetic dominant. (Most people become parasympathetic dominant after their adrenal glands have become exhausted.)

As we've discussed, the autonomic nervous system is a principal regulator of body function. It's composed of the sympathetic and parasympathetic systems. The sympathetic system is designed for "fight or flight" and thus favors the muscular system and the body's ability to respond physically with increased performance in threatening situations. Its balancing counterpart, the parasympathetic nervous system, is designed for promoting digestion, keeping the mucus membranes moist (think vaginal lubrication in your mate!) and promoting day-to-day management of the internal workings of the body.

Sympathetic types tend to have high energy, aggressive personalities, weak digestion, dry skin and excellent concentration. They tend to be tall, thin, have narrow shoulders, wider hips and are commonly underweight. They build muscle easily and tend to crave carbohydrates. They are prone to osteoporosis, infections, angina, heart disease, cancer, acute arthritis, diabetes, gallbladder attacks, ulcers, glaucoma and gingivitis (inflamed gums).

Excessive sympathetic responses fatigue the pituitary, thyroid, adrenals and testes. I would like to mention that there is no real significant anatomical or nervous tissue component difference between the two systems; the difference is the bio-chemicals that are involved.

Parasympathetic types tend to be slow, deliberate and cautious about their feelings. They are usually emotionally stable and able to make friends easily. They sometimes have low motivation, a tendency for allergies and asthma, low blood sugar, skin problems and poor concentration. They are generally wider built, with broad shoulders and good strength and endurance. Often their pupils are constricted, the membranes of the mouth and nose are moist with excess saliva/mucus, their heart rate is slow and their blood pressure is low.

Parasympathetic dominance promotes osteoarthritis and calcification of soft tissues, as with cataracts, kidney stones, calcific bursitis, heel and bone spurs, hardening of the arteries and heart valves. From the standpoint of whole-body health, it is important to have balance in the autonomic nervous system. This allows for optimal metabolism and digestion. The glands involved in the function of the parasympathetic nervous system include the pituitary, thyroid and adrenal tissues. It's important to note that the parasympathetic nervous system promotes digestion and is also responsible for relaxation and sleep.

A healthy person is able to appropriately engage the parasympathetic and the sympathetic nervous systems at the necessary times with great benefit to body, mind and spirit. The parasympathetic and sympathetic nervous systems must be regulated to the precise degree in the correct timing, reacting to the circumstance at hand. In certain situations, an individual may need to be nearly 100 percent parasympathetic (while eating dinner, for example); at other times, 40 percent parasympathetic and 60 percent sympathetic (for instance, drinking water while taking a walk with your spouse) would be the requirement. And, less often, 100 percent sympathetic would best suit the situation (immediately following a natural disaster, let's say). Environmental circumstances determine the needed percentages. When both systems are working in correct balance, it's like a profitable partnership! When one or the other becomes dominant, the nervous system becomes a hindrance rather than a help in accomplishing daily tasks.

If, as you read this, you are becoming more determined to engage or disengage your sympathetic or parasympathetic systems through willpower, think again. The balance between them is an unconscious act that functions more perfectly only when you make conscious choices toward good health.

ARE YOU SYMPATHETIC OR PARASYMPATHETIC DOMINANT?

Below is a simple screen to determine which category you fall into. Look over the following groups of symptoms and mark the ones that describe you. You may recognize yourself in both groups; however, you will generally score higher in one or the other.

PERSONAL HEALTH ASSESSMENT

Sympathetic Dominant		
☐ Acid foods upset	☐ High gag reflex	☐ Reduced appetite
☐ Often feel chilled	☐ Unable to relax; startle easily	☐ Frequent cold sweats
☐ "Lump" in throat	☐ Extremities cold, clammy	☐ Fever easily raised
☐ Dry mouth, eyes, nose	☐ Irritated by strong light	☐ Neuralgia-like pains
☐ Pulse quickens after meal	☐ Urine amount reduced	☐ Staring, blink little
☐ Nervous tension, unable to calm oneself	☐ Heart pounds after retiring	☐ Frequent sour stomach

Parasympathetic Dominant		
☐ Joint stiffness after rising	☐ Always seem hungry; feel "lightheaded" often	☐ Difficulty swallowing
☐ Muscle, leg, toe cramps at night	☐ Rapid Digestion	☐ Constipation, diarrhea alternating
☐ Nervous stomach, cramps	☐ Frequent vomiting	☐ Slow starter
☐ Eyes or nose watery	☐ Frequent hoarseness	☐ Not easily chilled
☐ Eyes blink often	☐ Irregular breathing	☐ Perspire easily
☐ Eyelids swollen, puffy	☐ Pulse slow; feels "irregular"	☐ Poor circulation Sensitive to cold
☐ Indigestion soon after meals	☐ Little gag reflex	☐ Subject to colds, asthma, bronchitis

If you marked several in the first list, you would tend to be sympathetic dominant. Specific treatments determined by a qualified health care provider may be helpful depending on the symptoms you're experiencing.

If you scored high in the second group of symptoms, you are most likely parasympathetic dominant. From my clinical observation, patients in this group were formerly sympathetic dominant but they fed their cravings and body signals with stimulants, such as caffeine and sugar, leading to adrenal exhaustion and many of the symptoms in the Sympathetic Dominance Table. The more symptoms an individual checks in the assessment above, the more of an autonomic imbalance they tend to have. I've found this to be the case regardless of which group they fall into. Eventually, they'll experience multiple symptoms from both groups as their nervous system function degrades more and more over time.

Most patients experiencing the sexual dysfunction rampant in our fast-paced culture fall into the sympathetic-dominant nervous system category. Men who are persistently stressed have difficulty achieving and maintaining erections. Stress results in sympathetic dominance, the adrenal excitation creates fatigue and he reaches for artificial stimulants, leading to continued sympathetic dominance. At the end of a stress-filled day, a couple may go to make love with each other and the whole vicious cycle has robbed their bodies of the ability to have spontaneous, enjoyable sex—the one thing that has the potential to bring the most relaxation and pleasure to their day!

WHAT YOU CAN DO

As we've discussed throughout this book, medication can help you achieve and maintain an erection, but it adds a number of sobering side effects to an already fatigued body. Medication also ignores the other body warning signals of autonomic nervous system imbalance. Equally troubling is the prospect of taking medication to correct every symptom experienced; imagine what a potentially fatal drug cocktail that would be! No, treatment does not have to be as complicated as a medicine cabinet that resembles the local drugstore. You have the power to make small changes that will return your body to a wonderfully balanced state. Of course, it's best to have the assistance of a knowledgeable health care provider as you take steps toward living a drugless lifestyle.

If you checked multiple boxes on the symptom list and suspect that your adrenal gland function is compromised, now is the time to make some changes. We learned in the first paragraph of this chapter that your body is a complex, interdependent network of systems whose functions impact one another in multiple ways. This is excellent news, because small changes will have a profound effect throughout your whole body. As you care for your body, it will pay you back with great health, great energy, great enjoyment and great sex.

YOUR ADRENAL GLANDS – ACTION STEPS

☐ A key to long-term adrenal health is adequate rest. Make whatever changes are necessary in your schedule to assure eight hours of sleep each night. Limit TV and computer time before bed to allow your mind and body time to relax without stimulation. Sleep in a cool, dark room; cover the small lights from your alarm clock and appliances. If you are experiencing adrenal exhaustion, make arrangements that allow you to sleep until between 7 a.m. and 9 a.m. each morning, as this is when your body is ending deep sleep and the restoration of cortisol levels for another day; the natural increase of cortisol levels is a part of the stimulus that wakes you naturally. Adrenal fatigue and exhaustion with concurrent unnatural low cortisol levels is, in fact, one of the reasons why some people have to literally drag themselves out of bed in the morning when their clock goes off.

☐ Gymnema is an excellent herb that reduces the taste for sweet items; take one to three caplets daily. Add more protein to your diet. Protein helps stabilize the rate your body burns energy and eliminates the extreme highs and lows that sugar induces. If you are consuming large amounts of nutritionally empty carbohydrates, your system will actually burn muscle to get the energy it needs to function. Limit protein to three to five ounces per serving so you do not get a compensatory insulin release, which can start a cascade of cravings for sweets.

☐ Avoid sweet fruits, especially bananas, raisins and grapes. Eat veggies as a snack with nuts, such as almonds or walnuts, plus sunflower seeds.

☐ If you crave salt (a common adrenal-fatigue symptom), consume Celtic Sea Salt®.

☐ Avoid supplementing DHEA, which can upset the delicate balance of hormones in your body. Instead, seek out a skilled health care provider to help you manage adrenal fatigue.

☐ Consume vitamin C-sourced foods. A delicious choice and one that is available year-round is a mixed green salad with vitamin

C–rich red, yellow and orange bell peppers. Vitamin C is an integral component of adrenal health. I do not encourage citrus because it tends to create an alkaline pH, commonly observed in females over 40 resulting in fibromyalgia.

☐ If you have low blood pressure, consider using a whole-food B-complex vitamin supplement. Again, you should consult an experienced health care provider during treatment.

☐ Get a tissue-hair mineral analysis to determine your adrenal health. If your adrenal function is stressed, this test will often reveal decreased sodium and potassium and increased aluminum. The test also determines other mineral levels and is useful in creating a treatment program.

☐ Complete saliva hormone testing to get a baseline of your endocrine and hormone systems' function. Free hormones are measured in saliva testing; protein-bound hormones in serum testing. Go to **www.druglessdoctor.com** under the Client Services/Testing Services link for details.

☐ Maca root–sourced products have successfully helped many of my male patients have increased libido.

14

PAUSE FOR A SECOND...

Andropause, the male version of menopause, is a relatively new concept. While male sex hormones may experience a slight decline with age, and though there are potential genetic and birth defect challenges as one gets older, men were designed to perform sexually and father children indefinitely. Amazingly, you would never know this by watching all the pharmaceutical advertisements for erectile dysfunction on American TV! Once again, unhealthy lifestyles complicate the normal decline of hormones during aging, bringing about a whole host of accompanying symptoms.

SUMMARY OF ANDROPAUSE

- Defined as a loss of androgen dominance in men.
- Caused by functional imbalances in the male hormone pathway wherein free testosterone declines 1-2 percent yearly.
- Testosterone is made from cholesterol and plays an important role in supporting the thyroid and healthy triglycerides. Cholesterol-lowering statin drugs are shown to reduce testosterone.
- Symptoms may include mood swings, depression, passivity and cynicism.

- Physical symptoms include muscle weakness, insulin resistance, high blood pressure, mid-body fat gain, blood sugar issues, osteoporosis and thin, dry skin.
- Sexual symptoms include decreased libido, erectile dysfunction and prostate/urinary problems.

CAUSES OF ANDROPAUSE

"Androgen," as mentioned in Chapter 2 on balancing male hormones, is the generic term for any natural or synthetic compound that stimulates or controls the development and maintenance of masculine characteristics by binding to androgen receptors. This includes the activity of the accessory male sex organs (the testes, epididymis and seminal vesicles) and the development of secondary male sex characteristics (such as facial hair, deepening of the voice, etc.).

Testosterone is secreted primarily in the testes of males and the ovaries of females, although small amounts are secreted by the adrenal glands. In both men and women, testosterone plays a key role in libido, energy levels, immunity and protection against osteoporosis. As discussed earlier in the book, an adult male, on average, produces 20 to 30 times the amount of testosterone an adult woman does.

A lot of the media coverage on the "aging baby boomers" states that menopause should be an easy transition in women and that andropause in men shouldn't even exist. But if that were the case, then why are so many 40- to 55-year-old patients dragging themselves into my office with the symptoms mentioned above? To be blunt, it's because too many people aren't serious about investing in their health. We plan for retirement, we plan for vacation, we plan for our children's college funds, but somehow the planning it takes to maintain a healthy body falls to the wayside. Think of your body as a bank account. You can put in deposits and create a base of "health wealth," or you can continually make withdrawals until you're finally forced to declare bankruptcy. Just walk around at any public function and you will see an overwhelming number of people with figurative "foreclosure" signs hovering over their heads. Obesity and hobbling are commonplace.

When men come into my office experiencing symptomatic andropause, I can almost always pinpoint two basic causes: 1) adrenal and thyroid burnout and/or 2) decreased liver function. The adrenal glands are designed to be your steroid hormone backup, and your thyroid keeps energy levels high. I have explained more about these challenges in Chapters 13 and 15 on the adrenal glands and thyroid, respectively. In this chapter, we'll focus on the major culprits in andropause challenges, beginning with stress.

STRESS

When stress levels are constantly high, they lead to impaired adrenal function. The nutrients for routine cellular function are being used to make cortisone to handle the stress, leaving very little to make testosterone. Cholesterol production is also diverted to make ever-increasing amounts of cortisone instead of being used for sex-based steroid hormones. The result? Symptomatic andropause.

Patients presenting these symptoms very often fit the same mold. Their work and personal commitments are extremely demanding, occasionally to the point of physical collapse. The women experiencing a difficult menopause have typically reached a point of hormonal exhaustion anywhere between 40 and 50 years old, sometimes even earlier. These ladies are raising children, some even grandchildren, caring for the household, working and contributing to the family finances and possibly caring for one or more elderly parents. Men, you statistically do not have it any easier. Are you feeling trapped by family finances into working extremely long hours at a job that may include shift changes, business travel and demanding clients? On top of all the responsibilities, both men and women are juggling marriage, child rearing, friendships and commitments to church and community organizations. It's no wonder everyone is exhausted and taking antidepressants! Add to this confusion the challenges of mixed and blended households and you can understand why patients come staggering into my office looking for help.

A reminder about financial responsibility is warranted here. As I said in Chapter 2, your earning power will never satisfy your yearning desire. That is, no matter how much money you bring in, there will always be one more toy that you'd like to own. I know there are fixed expenses and important investments, but you should do everything you can to minimize your consumption of, and desire for, material possessions. Each new thing you purchase translates into a certain number of hours worked to pay for it. That work and added stress takes a toll on your health.

ALCOHOL AND DRUG USE, PRESCRIPTION MEDICATION

Compounding the stress of daily life is the excessive use of alcohol along with prescription and recreational drugs. Alcohol puts added strain on liver function. Escaping the pressures of life by consuming alcohol and drugs is a slippery slope that can lead to addiction. Over 50 percent of insured Americans are on at least one prescription medication, with many more Americans regularly taking multiple prescriptions each day. As we have discussed, these medications treat the symptom while ignoring the root cause, and of course most, if not all, come with their own set of deleterious side effects. Therefore, make the first solution you reach for a natural one.

POOR NUTRITION LEADING TO STRESS ON THE LIVER

Today's typical diet is filled with sugar. The negative effects of sugar are actually more powerful than the positive attributes of wholesome food and quality supplements. If there were only one change I could influence you to make, it would be to minimize your consumption of sugar and sugar substitutes. Many more tips on that in Chapter 17 on the Page Fundamental Diet. Processed foods have been stripped of nutrients that are absolutely essential for good health, yet they've become a staple in our diets. We're also consuming higher and higher levels of toxic chemicals, which, as you have discovered, stress the liver. If changes aren't made, both men and women will suffer from the resulting general poor health, including the loss of sexual desire and ability to perform. I can't emphasize enough that your diet should be full of whole foods that provide the nutrients your body needs to maintain good health, and you should be able to avoid andropause altogether.

INSUFFICIENT IODINE

A leading culprit in symptomatic andropause is insufficient iodine. We have discussed this before and will cover it more in Chapter 15 on the thyroid, but it bears a mention here because of its role in andropause. I have consistently observed symptoms of urinary urgency in men with low levels of iodine. Iodine supplementation can help. Therefore, a quality source of sea minerals that contains iodine would be an excellent adjunct to your daily food intake; Celtic Sea Salt® is an example of a mineral that can be applied liber- ally to your meals. Kelp and sea vegetables are also a fine source of iodine; I have recommended up to nine kelp tablets a day for my male patients. Kelp supplementation, by the way, also assists the body in binding and releasing toxins. As a reminder, you should avoid using hot tubs and pools with bromine and chlorine, as these chemical compounds are antagonistic to iodine and compete for iodine receptors. Iodine supplements will also be beneficial if you suffer from dry eyes and chronic sinus challenges. Additionally, my experience with patients has shown that iodine decreases PSA readings in men who experience prostate challenges.

INSUFFICIENT ZINC

A zinc deficiency can also be responsible for symptomatic andropause. As we've discussed, sugar, stress and consuming wheat and soy products all deplete zinc. Memory loss, slow healing, white spots on the nails and impaired insulin function can be precipitated by a zinc deficiency. I also generally see a diminished sense of taste and smell in patients lacking zinc. Zinc is a critical ingredient in prostate function in men.

ESTROGEN SATURATION

An overabundance of estrogen—in men, women and children—can in many cases create symptomatic hormonal challenges. To determine if you suffer from estrogen saturation, check your abdomen, arms and legs for those small, raised, cherry-colored bumps called "cherry hemangiomas." For men, these can translate into prostate issues and altered libido. For a review on ways to combat estrogen saturation, reread Chapters 2 and 8 on the male hormones and the liver, respectively.

Aging men shouldn't be assigned to decreased libido and erectile challenges. These "-pause" symptoms can be avoided by making daily investments into your health bank account. The dividends of maintaining "health wealth" include energy, stamina, passion for life, muscle strength and a consistent sex life well into old age, in addition to the peace of mind that comes with knowing you will continue to have good health and wonderful golden years.

PAUSE FOR A SECOND – ACTION STEPS

☐ Are you experiencing any of the symptoms of andropause?

☐ Sit down with your calendar and identify activities that can be removed to minimize stress.

☐ Limit or eliminate alcohol consumption and discontinue illegal drug use. Consult with a natural health care professional about ways to treat high blood pressure, cholesterol, etc., without the use of prescription drugs. Don't stop taking these medications without the approval of your doctor.

☐ Eliminate sugar, sugar substitutes and processed foods from your diet. Instead, eat a diet rich in whole foods and organic meats. Consume three to five ounces of protein with each meal. Consult Chapter 17 on the Page Fundamental Diet Plan for meal ideas.

☐ For optimal hormonal production, take one tablespoon of flax oil per 100 pounds of your body weight.

☐ Iodine supplementation is critical for long-term health. I encourage my patients to take up to 12 mg of an iodine/iodide combination daily. Before working your way up to that level of supplementation, you should have either a urine iodine loading test or a urine iodine level assessment to determine iodine levels in your system.

☐ Reread Chapters 2 and 8 on the male hormones and liver for ways to avoid estrogen saturation.

☐ Tribulus is an herb that will help increase the production of testosterone in men. My patients routinely take a maca root–based product along with tribulus.

☐ Saliva hormone testing is an excellent assessment for evaluating your hormone levels. This test is available by going to **www.druglessdoctor.com** under the Client Services/Testing Services link.

☐ Exercise a minimum of 30 minutes daily. Incorporate both aerobic and muscle strength training.

15

THE OTHER 'ROID

"**C**old hands, warm heart" is an old cliché, but having cold hands can be an awkward warning sign of thyroid problems. Your thyroid gland is located in the middle of the throat and is an important component of the endocrine system. It has many roles, including regulating body temperature and ensuring that you will have warm hands *and* a warm heart! The thyroid regulates metabolism (including bowel and colon function) and also works closely with the adrenal glands to provide energy. Sexual desire and ability are closely related to and affected by thyroid function.

In our fast-paced society, it's not uncommon for both men and women to experience thyroid and adrenal gland exhaustion, resulting in decreased energy and lowered sexual desire. Low thyroid function is one of the most common diagnoses among new patients who come to me seeking natural treatment for health issues. They feel out of control and overwhelmed, and few consider that their problems may be caused by decreased thyroid function. Many are taking Synthroid®, a common prescription medication for low thyroid activity, and are beginning to question its validity in the face of more natural treatment methods. Others are being pressured to start thyroid medication and are hesitant to do so due to negative side effects.

COMMON LOW THYROID BODY SIGNALS

Look over the following list of symptoms and see if you recognize any in your own life:

☐ obesity

☐ fatigue

☐ thinning hair

☐ widely spaced teeth

☐ high cholesterol

☐ cold hands and feet

☐ yellow teeth

☐ feeling chilled in the morning

☐ constipation

☐ emotional distress

☐ high estrogen levels (swollen prostate, enlarged breasts)

☐ leg cramps at night

☐ morning headaches that wear off as the day progresses

☐ thinning of the outer eyebrows

☐ dry skin

Feeling Chilled and Having Cold Extremities

The thyroid acts like a thermostat to regulate body temperature. Many patients complain of being chilled in the fall and winter. If you find yourself wearing winter pajamas all year round, your thyroid may be suspect. If you experience feeling chilled and have cold hands and feet, you may want to limit your intake of cruciferous foods, including broccoli, cauliflower and cabbage. For the general public these are excellent sources of nutrients and fiber, but

I've found they sometimes impair thyroid function and should be avoided at least for a while. Once body temperature is regulated, you may add them back into your diet, either steaming or sautéing the vegetables. It's not necessary to eat them raw as some health journals suggest, and cooking them slightly might actually deter some of the digestive challenges they often present. Soy products should be avoided since they are antagonistic to thyroid function, as well as for the other reasons stated elsewhere in this book. To ensure proper fiber in your diet during this time, consume green beans, zucchini, peppers, asparagus and steamed carrots. Deb and I enjoy a mixed green salad for lunch almost every day, avoiding iceberg lettuce, which has little, if any, nutritional value.

A more significant concern created by subpar thyroid activity affecting men and women is persistent elevated cholesterol that is unresponsive to the accepted dietary modifications of limited red meat and dairy. As the thyroid grows stressed and exhausted, it loses the ability to normally regulate body metabolism; the consistent finding I see in my practice is a seemingly "idiopathic" elevated LDL cholesterol level that causes the most astute practitioner to scratch their head. I've discovered that this elusive condition is often caused by a lack of iodine in the diet, which is discussed in more detail later in this chapter. As we've discussed, toxic chemical compounds such as bromine, fluorine and chlorine compete with iodine, further impairing thyroid function. Excessive intake of processed foods full of partially hydrogenated fat (trans fat) impedes liver function, in turn limiting the hormones the thyroid needs to regulate cholesterol levels.

Constipation

Because the thyroid has an impact on bowel and colon activity, its impairment often results in constipation. Many people choose to treat constipation with laxatives. While laxatives may work temporarily, it's easy to become dependent on them for bowel movements and continue ignoring your body's cry for healthy habits. The correct natural method to treat this condition is to increase water and fiber consumption. I often encourage my patients to allow time for rest and relaxation in the morning, which generally leads to a bowel movement.

Emotional Distress

Many people seeking psychiatric treatment for emotional issues are often suffering from impaired thyroid function. Stress has an incredibly large impact on the thyroid and adrenal glands, causing fatigue and anxiety.

I've actually treated patients who experienced panic attacks as their wedding approached—both brides and grooms! One patient ended up in the emergency room three days before the wedding. After consulting him, I determined the anxiety attack was in response to an overdose of sugar. This sweet culprit robs the body of nutrients needed for enzyme and hormone function. (I always felt kind of bad for this couple. If the wedding itself was so stressful, I can't imagine what the rest of the marriage will be like!)

If you have chronic emotional distress, you should have a proper thyroid assessment by an experienced health care professional familiar with endocrine function and the natural treatment of such. I see more and more young patients who are currently taking two different prescription antidepressants. This is a sobering trend among young people who are being medicated and overmedicated at a crucial time in their lives as they are starting careers, marriages and families. They would be better served by a thyroid malfunction diagnosis and natural treatment of their symptoms rather than masking the problem with prescription drugs. Please note, however, that if you are currently taking any medications for emotional distress issues, you should not discontinue them until talking with your doctor. Tyrosine and iodine combine to create thyroid hormone. Tyrosine is an amino acid that is clinically proven to aid in the treatment of depression. Adding tyrosine to my patients' treatment has consistently benefited those dealing with emotional challenges.

I don't intend to deliberately pinpoint women in a discussion of emotional distress, but I do treat far more women than men for depression and depression-related syndromes. I believe this is simply based on the fact that women have a larger puzzle of hormones (including iodine deficiencies) in their endocrine balance sheet than men do. Men primarily need iodine for thyroid and testes/prostate function, while women need it for proper function of all their hormones and for the thyroid, breasts and ovaries. It is true, however, that the health of every cell in both men and women is impacted by iodine.

I generally consult with men, often between 35 and 40 years old, who are really hard pressed to take antidepressants "just to take the edge off." And then there is the new trend of prescribing anti-psychotic and antidepressants to the youth of America. In 2009 alone, 10 million prescriptions were recommended for "kids" under 20. This, from my perspective, is only going to continue. Our children are bombarded by toxins from birth, compounding their potential to have thyroid challenges from the beginning. Growing pains, unexplained fevers and leg cramps at night are common body signals of thyroid problems.

Other possible factors in depression include insufficient omega-3 oils, lack of minerals and a low supply of B vitamins. Many doctors are quick to prescribe medications, but they come with the unfortunate side effect of diminished sexual appetite, among many others. Once again, the symptoms are treated, the cause is masked and negative side effects wreak their own havoc on the body and the marriage or relationship. Increasing thyroid function with natural methods is so simple and successful—I don't know why anyone wouldn't want to give it a try when the benefits are so quickly experienced.

Managing a Morning Headache

Headaches in the morning can be a real . . . PAIN! When I treat a patient who wakes up with morning headaches, I always ask first what they ate before going to sleep. The most common answer is something full of sugar, even a food as seemingly harmless as a sweet dried fruit. During the night, the thyroid and adrenal processing of sugar is decreased, resulting in increased blood sugar and voila!—a morning headache.

Fatigue

The thyroid's role in energy is like the gas pedal on a car. No gas means no energy. While fatigue can occur at any age, I especially see people over 40 suffering from this condition.

Coarse Hair That Falls Out, Thinning of the Hair and Eyebrows, Widely Spaced and/or Yellow Teeth

Minerals affect thyroid gland productivity. When the thyroid is stressed or does not receive adequate nutritional building blocks, mineral absorption decreases. The results vary, from changes in hair texture, thinning of hair on the head and eyebrows, to changes in teeth placement. Yellowed teeth are also common in patients with a sluggish thyroid as calcium uptake is impaired and teeth become discolored.

THE ROLE OF IODINE IN THYROID FUNCTION

Iodine is one of the major components the thyroid uses to create thyroid hormone. Unfortunately, the amount of iodine most people have available for cellular function is largely inadequate. The World

Health Organization has said that 72 percent of the world's population does not have enough iodine. The iodized salt purchased at conventional grocery stores also generally contains aluminum and dextrose for anti-caking purposes, and therefore I don't encourage its use. Sodium chloride (table salt) can actually create challenges with normal thyroid function. Instead, switch to hand-harvested Celtic Sea Salt®. It's a great source of easy-to-assimilate minerals, including iodine.

I also want to remind you about the anti-thyroid compounds we've discussed in other chapters that can interfere with the normal receptor sites for iodine. These include bromine, fluorine and chlorine. Bromine replaced iodine as a conditioner in bread in the early 1960s. Commercial white bread products, consumed in great quantities in America, can actually create thyroid distress. Bromine is found in certain beverages including soda and sports drinks and is an ingredient in some antidepressants. The irony is sobering: that psycho-active medications commonly used to treat depression can actually promote it as bromine interferes with iodine metabolism.

Fluorine is put in most municipalities' water supplies and is also a common oral application at well-meaning dental offices. Deb and I personally do not drink tap water nor do we receive fluoride treatments, and we haven't had a cavity in decades. So what's our source of fluoride? Nope, not toothpaste. It's carrots! The same is true for both of our sons, who were born in the 1980s. You can continue to have strong teeth, gums and enamel very easily by eliminating the number one cause—stop sugar.

Chlorine is a little-known but very common anti-iodine compound. If you use a dishwasher detergent that contains this toxic chemical and happen to breathe it in, you're getting your share of chlorine. The same is true of the steam you inhale while taking a shower in chlorinated water. For this reason, I encourage the use of chlorine-free dishwasher soap as well as the installation of a de-chlorinating showerhead. You should also limit the amount of time spent in hot tubs and swimming pools. We've seen patients who suffer from chronic leg cramps as a result of swimming and exercising in bromine- and chlorine-saturated pools. The sweetener Splenda®, which is sourced from sugar, also stresses the thyroid due to the chlorine in its composition.

I can't overstate the vital role iodine plays in the production of hormones affecting sexuality. Men's PSA (prostate assessment) levels lower when their diet is supplemented with adequate iodine and they are monitored by the urine iodine loading test. (See Chapter 9 on cancer.)

The Barnes Thyroid Temperature Test is a simple way to screen whether your thyroid is possibly not functioning as it should. Place a shaken-down or battery-operated thermometer by your bedside some evening. The next morning, upon waking, place the stem of thermometer in your armpit for 10 minutes. (This should be done even before getting out of bed and going to the bathroom.) The temperature reading should be 97.8° Fahrenheit or higher; if it's lower, you should focus on adding a source of iodine to your diet. This can be in the form of kelp, sea vegetables, ocean seafood or Celtic Sea Salt®. Repeat this simple self-assessment at least monthly while supplementing with iodine-based foods. If your temperature hasn't changed, seek a natural health care provider who has experience treating thyroid conditions with appropriate supplementation and diet modifications. Tissue-hair mineral analysis may also be an important step in the diagnosis of a thyroid-related problem.

Your health care provider may also check your TSH, T3 and T4 levels to determine if thyroid hormone levels are sufficient. Low levels of T3 and T4 often suggest a deficiency of both tyrosine and iodine. The treatment for high TSH often includes a form of cell therapy with an animal tissue source of thyroid DNA. A low TSH reading may suggest the pituitary gland is in need of some assistance. Occasionally these tests come back with normal levels even though a patient is experiencing all the common symptoms of thyroid malfunction such as cold extremities, constipation and high cholesterol. If the tests are within normal range and you suspect your thyroid is the cause, seek a health care provider who is open to natural forms of treatment.

A diet full of nutrients that positively impact thyroid health includes flax oil, beets, plenty of protein, sea vegetables and deep ocean fish. Fruits should be limited. You may not notice changes in your thyroid tests for up to two years upon initiating a natural protocol, but you would be wise to pursue a natural treatment, as thyroid medication does not cure the problem nor assist the body in calcium metabolism.

THYROID – ACTION STEPS

- ☐ Browse the symptom list and choose one or two areas of thyroid health that can be improved. If you have multiple symptoms, commit to making at least one diet or lifestyle change each week.

- ☐ Have your urine iodine levels assessed, and supplement accordingly.

- ☐ Avoid exposure to bromine, fluorine and chlorine. Obtain a water purifier and a shower de-chlorinator.

- ☐ Have your TSH, T3 and T4 thyroid blood tests assessed.

- ☐ Avoid consuming soy foods, as they deplete iodine.

16

SWEETENERS: "DR. BOB APPROVED" AND NOT APPROVED

Most of my patients have questions about sugar and "natural" sugar alternatives. Increased sugar consumption is a contributing factor to behavioral challenges, and it is a leading cause of many other health conditions as well. Because you might have chronic sinusitis, migraines, headaches or back pain, it is very important for you to understand why you need to be a label reader.

The average American consumes *149 pounds* of refined sugar each year! If your body were to convert this, it would add 79 pounds of fat. By calculating the amount of sugar that comes from soda consumption, it is easy to see why our children are in a diminished state of health. Most Americans eat too much refined sugar, which travels through your mouth and stomach tissues right to your bloodstream. This wreaks havoc on your blood sugar levels and your immune system.

Our human instinct to seek sweeteners is so strong that an unborn baby will make swallowing motions when its mother is injected with a sweetener. This intense instinct for sweeteners causes us to seek out sweet breast milk. Even in adulthood, sugar continues to be a common craving. Have you had something sweet to eat within the last 24-48 hours? If not, do you plan on having something sweet very shortly?

WHAT IS SUGAR'S BIG APPEAL?

Sweet foods have become hopelessly intertwined with pleasure and euphoria. These foods are alluring, symbolizing reward or comfort. After a hard day at work or school, devouring a candy bar seems to be a valid reward (or a survival mechanism). Sugar causes our brains to release endorphins, a "feel good" chemical. Yet, it is not white sugar or derivatives that your body wants—it wants complex carbohydrates that are as whole as breast milk.

All sugars are not created equal. Some would say there is no differentiation between natural or refined sugars because our bodies use both for energy. I disagree! Sugars can be either simple or complex carbohydrates. Naturally occurring sugars are almost always complex carbohydrates; white (or refined) sugars are almost always simple carbohydrates. Complex carbohydrates (like those in beans, fruit, vegetables and whole grains) are made of long chains of simple sugar. Your body digests them more slowly and provides your blood with a more balanced sugar supply. Whatever sugar your body doesn't immediately need is stored in your liver as glycogen, an energy reserve.

> White sugar is a human invention, not a gift from nature. In 1795, Louisiana farmers devised a cheaper way to granulate sugar on a large scale, which made white sugar available to the masses.

Complex carbohydrates give you all the energy you need. When you are looking for something to satisfy your sweet tooth, however, turn to natural sweeteners like rice and barley malt syrups that are

50 percent complex carbohydrates. The human body's digestive enzymes break these two types of sugars down to glucose, a sugar that the body uses for energy. The difference between simple and complex carbohydrates is how quickly each enters the bloodstream and how each affects insulin in blood sugar levels—a real key, I believe, to why we have major problems with obesity in our society today. When your insulin level skyrockets from the rush of sugar found in nearly every item in the grocery and convenience stores, the body responds by stopping the use of body fat for energy, instead storing it for use on another day that rarely presents itself since we eat an average of one-half a teaspoon of sugar every half hour!

Here is an example of the vicious cycle of refined sugar cravings:

First: Energy rush. Simple sugars go directly into your bloodstream, giving you a temporary high.

Second: Pancreatic panic begins. You may be on your "high," feeling good, but your high blood sugar is causing your pancreas to scream, "DANGER!" As a result, there is an enormous response from your pancreas, dumping huge amounts of insulin into your blood, bringing your blood sugar level down again.

Third: This rush of insulin causes a fast crash. Blood sugar levels swing too low too fast, leading to the sugar blues (leaving you with fatigue and irritability and perhaps a hyperactive response).

Fourth: Your energy crash will stimulate your need for another sugar rush to elevate your energy to normalcy. You are trapped in a sugar rush cycle.

THE HAZARDS OF EATING SUGAR

There are long-term health hazards associated with refined sugar, including a depletion of your body's essential minerals and B vitamins. Refined sugar is actually a stripped carbohydrate. When sugar cane—the raw material for sugar—is turned into refined sugar, it is depleted of minerals and nutritional elements. Eating a depleted or stripped carbohydrate forces your body to use its own vitamins and minerals for digestion. Over time, excessive consumption of refined sugars can lead to nutritional deficiencies and serious problems like osteoporosis, gum disease and arthritis.

Your body can't produce enough digestive enzymes without the right balance of minerals and B vitamins. Compensating for your sweet tooth by consuming additional healthy foods may be a losing battle since your body is no longer digesting or assimilating food efficiently. This is another real challenge for children who are hyperactive, since they are already consuming food that is nutritionally stripped.

NOTICE: Eating sugar puts stress on digestion.
Poor digestion can lead to allergies.
Sugar consumption results in poor health.

SWEETENERS TO AVOID

What about other refined sugars? Following are a variety of sugars and sugar substitutes to avoid:

Brown sugar is simply refined sugar that is sprayed with molasses to make it appear more whole. Turbinado sugar gives the illusion of health but is just one step away from white sugar. Turbinado is made from 95 percent sucrose (table sugar). It skips only the final filtration stage of sugar refining, resulting in little difference in nutritional value.

Corn syrup or **high-fructose corn syrup (HFCS)** is found everywhere. It is used in everything from bouillon cubes to spaghetti sauce and even in some "natural" juices. Corn syrup processed from cornstarch is almost as sweet as refined sugar and is absorbed quickly by your blood. Corn-derived sweeteners pose other problems too: They often contain high levels of pesticide residues that are genetically modified and are common allergy producers. This is a cheap and plentiful sweetener often used in soft drinks, candy and baked goods. Corn syrup is very similar to refined sugar in composition as well as effect. I would avoid high-fructose corn syrup and maltodextrin, both of which are sourced from corn.

Aspartame, a common synthetic sweetener, affects the nervous system and brain in a very negative way. Aspartame is made from two proteins, or amino acids, which give it its super sweetness. Aspartame has many harmful effects: behavior changes in children, headaches, dizziness, epileptic-like seizures and bulging of the eyes, to name a few. Aspartame is an "excitotoxin," a substance that over-stimulates neurons and causes them to die suddenly (as though they were excited to death). One of the last steps of aspartame metabolism is formaldehyde. The next time you consume diet soda, think. You are literally embalming yourself.

Splenda®, a **sucralose**-based artificial sweetener, is marketed as being safer than aspartame because it is sourced from sugar. But, beware, Splenda® is basically chlorinated sugar! I highly suggest avoiding it.

Sucrose is found in white sugar. Sucrose requires very little digestion and provides instant energy followed by plummeting blood sugar levels. It causes the entire body stress.

Glucose is also called dextrose. When combined with sucrose, glucose subjects your blood sugar to the same ups and downs. In whole-food form—in starches like beans and whole grain breads, which are also rich in soluble fiber—glucose takes longer to digest, resulting in more balanced energy.

Sorbitol, Mannitol & Xylitol are synthetic sugar alcohols. Although these can cause less of an insulin jump in glucose to sugar, many people suffer gastric distress. You see these sugars listed as ingredients in foods.

Unrefined cane juice is sugarcane in crystal form—nothing more, nothing less. Unrefined cane juice is brown and granulated, contains 85 percent to 96.5 percent sucrose and, when arid, retains all of sugarcane's vitamins, minerals and other nutrients. Cane juice has a slightly stronger flavor and less intense sweetness than white sugar. In health food stores, be alert for sugars disguised as "evaporated cane juice" or "cane juice crystals." These can still cause problems, regardless of what the health food store manager tells you.

Crystalline fructose is a refined simple sugar that has the same molecular structure as fruit sugar. It's almost twice as sweet as white sugar and is released into the bloodstream slower than sucrose. Extra sugar gets stored in your liver as glycogen.

Agave is often reported as a "healthy" sugar alternative, though I would not personally use it. It is often labeled as "natural" and "organic" but often is highly processed in a laboratory. Use caution and read the label of any particular product you're considering consuming to see what may have been added.

STAR SWEETENERS:
THE BEST OF THE "NATURALS"

Become sugar savvy! The term "natural," as applied to sweeteners, can mean many things. The sweeteners recommended below will provide you with steady energy because they take a long time to digest. Natural choices offer rich flavors, vitamins and minerals, without the ups and downs of refined sugars.

Brown rice syrup: Your bloodstream absorbs this balanced syrup, high in maltose and complex carbohydrates, slowly and steadily. Brown rice syrup is a natural for baked goods and hot drinks: It adds subtle sweetness and a rich, butterscotch-like flavor. To get sweetness from starchy brown rice, the magic ingredients are enzymes, but the actual process varies depending on the syrup manufacturer. "Malted" syrups use whole, sprouted barley to create a balanced sweetener. Choose these syrups to make tastier muffins and cakes. Cheaper, sweeter rice syrups use isolated enzymes and are a bit harder on blood sugar levels. For a healthy treat, drizzle gently heated rice syrup over popcorn to make natural caramel corn. Store in a cool, dry place.

Barley malt syrup: As mentioned above, this sweetener is made much like rice syrup, but it uses sprouted barley to turn grain starches into a complex sweetener that is digested slowly. Use barley malt syrup to add molasses-like flavor and light sweetness to beans, cookies, muffins and cakes. Store in a cool, dry place.

Amasake is an ancient, oriental whole grain sweetener made from cultured brown rice. It has a thick, pudding-like consistency. Baked goods benefit from amasake's subtle sweetness, moisture and leavening power.

Stevia is a sweet South American herb that has been used safely for centuries by many cultures. Extensive scientific studies back up these ancient claims to safety. However, the FDA has approved it only when labeled as a dietary supplement, not as a sweetener. Advocates consider stevia to be one of the healthiest sweeteners as well as a tonic to heal the skin. Stevia is 150 to 400 times sweeter than white sugar, has no calories and can actually regulate blood sugar levels. Unrefined stevia has a molasses-like flavor; refined stevia (popular in Japan) has less flavor and nutrients.

Fruit Sweet®: This brand-name sweetener is a combination of pear and pineapple juice concentrates containing fruit sugars, mostly fructose, which in whole foods like this and in whole fruit balance energy, unlike refined sugar. Fruit Sweet® can also be used for baking.

Whole fruit: For baking, try fruit purees, dried fruit and cooked fruit sauces or butters. The less water remaining in a fruit, the more concentrated its flavor and sugar content. You'll find fiber and naturally balanced nutrients in whole fruits like apples, bananas and apricots. To add mild sweetness and moisture to baked goods, mix in the magic of mashed winter squashes, sweet potatoes and carrots!

Honey: It takes one bee an entire lifetime to produce a single tablespoon of honey from flower nectar. But that small amount goes a long way! Honey is mostly made of glucose and fructose and is up to twice as sweet as white sugar. Honey enters the bloodstream rapidly. Look for raw honey, which still contains some vitamins, minerals, enzymes and pollen. Honey varies in color (according to its flower source) and ranges in strength from mild clover to strong orange blossom. A benefit of eating honey produced in your geographical region is that it may reduce hay fever and allergy symptoms by bolstering your natural immunity. Note: Raw honey can lead to a toxic, sometimes fatal form of botulism in children under one. Limit honey consumption, as it gives similar results as sucrose.

Maltose is the primary sugar in brown rice and barley malt syrups. Maltose is a complex sugar that is digested slowly. It is the sugar with "staying power."

Maple Syrup: It takes about 10 gallons of maple sap to produce 1 gallon of maple syrup. Like honey, a little goes a long way. Maple syrup is roughly 65 percent sucrose and contains small amounts of trace minerals. Maple syrup has a rich taste and is absorbed fairly quickly into the bloodstream. Select real maple syrup that has no added corn syrup. Also, look for syrups that come from organic producers who don't use formaldehyde to prolong sap flow. Grade A syrups come from the first tapping; they range in color from light to dark amber. Grade B syrups come from the last tapping; they have more minerals and a stronger flavor and color.

Date sugar: This sweetener is made from dried, ground dates, is light brown and has a sugary texture. Date sugar retains many naturally occurring vitamins and minerals, is 65 percent sucrose and has a fairly rapid effect on blood sugar. Use it in baking instead of brown sugar but reduce your baking time or temperature in order to prevent premature browning. Store in a cool, dry place.

Concentrated fruit juice: All concentrates are not created equally. Highly refined juice sweeteners are labeled "modified." These sweeteners, similar to white sugar, have lost both their fruit flavor and their nutrients. Better choices are fruit concentrates that have been evaporated in a vacuum. These retain rich fruit flavors and aromas and many vitamins and minerals. Carefully read labels on cereal, cookie, jelly and beverage containers, then choose products with the highest percentage of real fruit juice. Beware of white grape juice concentrates that aren't organic; their pesticide residues can be high!

GLYCEMIC INDEX

The glycemic index is a measure of food's ability to raise blood glucose to variable degrees. The greater the blood glucose level, the greater the insulin response. Thus, we want to choose foods with low glycemic indices. See the table below. There are many specific benefits of consuming food with low glycemic indices:

1. Blood lipids are reduced in patients with high triglyceride levels.
2. Insulin secretion is reduced.

3. Overall blood-glucose control improves in insulin-dependent and noninsulin-dependent diabetic subjects.

4. There is a reduction in abnormal blood glucose, insulin and amino-acid levels in patients with liver disease.

5. Foods with low glycemic indices may enhance the feeling of being full and satisfied.

6. Foods with low glycemic indices may increase athletic performance.

GLYCEMIC INDICES OF FOODS

FOOD	GLYCEMIC INDEX
BREADS	
RYE (CRISPBREAD)	95
RYE (WHOLE MEAL)	89
RYE (WHOLE GRAIN, I.E. PUMPERNICKEL)	68
WHEAT (WHITE)	100
WHEAT (WHOLEMEAL)	100
PASTA	
MACARONI (WHITE, BOILED 5 MIN)	64
SPAGHETTI (BROWN, BOILED 15 MIN)	61
SPAGHETTI (WHITE, BOILED 15 MIN)	67
STAR PASTA (WHITE, BOILED 5 MIN)	54
CEREAL GRAINS	
BARLEY (PEARLED)	36
BUCKWHEAT	78
BULGUR	65
MILLET	103
RICE (BROWN)	81
RICE (INSTANT, BOILED 1 MIN)	65
RICE (PARBOILED, BOILED 5 MIN)	54
RICE (PARBOILED, BOILED 15 MIN)	68
RICE (POLISHED, BOILED 5 MIN)	58
RICE (POLISHED, BOILED 10—25 MIN)	81
RYE KERNELS	47
SWEET CORN	80
WHEAT KERNELS	63

FOOD	GLYCEMIC INDEX
BREAKFAST CEREALS	
"ALL BRAN"	74
CORNFLAKES	121
MUESLI	96
PORRIDGE OATS	89
PUFFED RICE	132
PUFFED WHEAT	110
SHREDDED WHEAT	97
"WEETEBIX"	108
COOKIES	
DIGESTIVE	82
OATMEAL	78
PLAIN CRACKERS (WATER BISCUITS)	100
"RICH TEA"	80
SHORTBREAD COOKIES	88
ROOT VEGETABLES	
POTATO (INSTANT)	120
POTATO (MASHED)	98
POTATO (NEW/WHITE BOILED)	80
POTATO (RUSSET, BAKED)	118
POTATO (SWEET)	70
YAM	74
LEGUMES	
BAKED BEANS (CANNED)	70
BENGAL GRAM DAL	12
BUTTER BEANS	46
CHICKPEAS (DRIED)	47
CHICKPEAS (CANNED)	60
FROZEN PEAS	74
GARDEN PEAS (FROZEN)	65
GREEN PEAS (CANNED)	50
GREEN PEAS (DRIED)	65
HARICOT BEANS (WHITE, DRIED)	54
KIDNEY BEANS (DRIED)	43
KIDNEY BEANS (CANNED)	74
LENTILS (GREEN, DRIED)	36

FOOD	GLYCEMIC INDEX
LENTILS (GREEN, CANNED)	74
LENTILS (RED, DRIED)	38
PINTO BEANS (DRIED)	80
PINTO BEANS (CANNED)	38
PEANUTS	15
SOYA BEANS (DRIED)	20
SOYA BEANS (CANNED)	22
FRUIT	
APPLE	52
APPLE JUICE	45
BANANA	84
GRAPES	62
GRAPEFRUIT	36
ORANGE	59
ORANGE JUICE	71
PEACH	40
PEAR	47
PLUM	34
RAISINS	93
SUGARS	
FRUCTOSE	26
GLUCOSE	138
HONEY	126
LACTOSE	57
MALTOSE	152
SUCROSE	83
DAIRY PRODUCTS	
CUSTARD	59
ICE CREAM	69
SKIM MILK	46
WHOLE MILK	44
YOGURT	52
SNACK FOODS	
CORN CHIPS	99
POTATO CHIPS	77

SUGAR SUBSTITUTION

Amount Indicates the Equivalent of 1 Cup of White Sugar

Sweetener	Amount	Liquid Reduction	Suggested Use
Honey	1/2 -2/3 cup	1/4 cup	All-purpose
Maple syrup	1/2 -3/4 cup	1/4 cup	Baking & desserts
Maple sugar	1/2 -1/3 cup	None	Baking & candies
Barley malt syrup	1 -1 1/2 cups	1/2 cup	Breads & baking
Rice syrup	1 -1/3 cups	1/2 cup	Baking & cakes
Date sugar	2/3 cup	None	Breads & baking
Fruit juice concentrate	1 cup	1/3 cup	All-purpose
Stevia	1 tsp/cup of water	1 cup	Baking

It is best to choose food with glycemic indices of 50–80. Foods in this range will give you the best chance to minimize exaggerated insulin responses. (Note: If you have a serious blood sugar regulation problem, such as diabetes or hypo-glycemia, see your health care practitioner to determine the type and amount of sweeteners your body can handle.)

SWEETENERS – ACTION STEPS

☐ Read labels—sugar is disguised by a variety of names. Its negative impact is the same regardless of what you call it.

☐ Avoid all artificial sweeteners. Your body needs to process them as it would any other foreign toxin.

☐ The names of alcohol sugars end in -ol. Though they have been promoted as safe alternatives, I would avoid them just like any other synthetic sweetener.

☐ Start your day without depending on pastries and items made with refined grains and sugars; eating these kinds of sugary carbs will start the roller coaster of high and low blood sugar and insulin levels.

☐ Take a whole-food chromium supplement, up to nine daily, to curtail your cravings for sugar.

NOTES

17

THE PAGE FUNDAMENTAL DIET PLAN

Patients always ask me what they should eat. It is probably one of the most common questions I get on a regular basis. One of my post-graduate training classes was a part of the curriculum from the International Foundation of Nutrition and Health (www.IFNH. org). They utilize the Page Diet protocol in their training.[1] I have adapted it in my office and have found it to be very logical, not to mention that it works for every aspect of health: restoration, weight loss, normalization of blood sugars and fats! Most people seem to focus on about eight or ten different foods and that is the extent of their diet. Most kids eat only about three foods—pizza, macaroni-and-cheese and chicken nuggets. And, of course, we cannot forget America's favorite vegetable—the French fry. Adult eating patterns are really not that much different from kids'. Few want to explore food choices beyond what they are used to.

While teaching one of my workshops, "The Drugless Approach to Female Hormones," I noticed a very conservatively dressed woman, whom I did not know, staring at me strangely the whole time I was speaking. I was beginning to think she was from some espionage group, there hoping to figure out what is in my "secret sauce," so to speak. I came to find out afterward that she had been staring at me in bewilderment after I had mentioned that beets can lower your cholesterol 40 percent and help to clean up the liver. She—unbelievable as it was—did not know what a beet was or looked like. WOW! I know that some of the foods and items discussed in this book are foreign to you. Do not get discouraged! I do not expect you to make immediate changes. Just try something new and be adventurous.

This diet plan is designed to assist your body in its ability to create and maintain "balanced body chemistry." Dr. Melvin Page's Phase I and Phase II diet is not only extremely helpful, but in many cases essential to controlling blood sugar imbalances as well as all other types of imbalanced body chemistry. At the famous Page Clinic, blood chemistry panels were done every three to four days on all patients. Dr. Page based his diet plan on the research of Drs. Price and Pottenger, who showed the relationship of diet to both physical and emotional health. The diet plan was proven true when blood chemistry panels of thousands of his patients normalized without any other intervention. Many of today's popular diets are based on Dr. Page's work. Dr. Page emphasized removing refined carbohydrates (such as sugar and processed flour) and pasteurized or processed cow's milk from the diet. In the following food list, notice that the percentage of carbohydrates is indicated. Dr. Page felt that it was not only important to eat quality proteins and fats, but quality carbohydrates as well.

The longer you are on this diet and the more closely you follow it, the easier it will be to stick to it. This will result in your feeling and looking much better than you did with your past eating habits. As you become healthier, your cravings for foods that aren't the best choices for you will actually diminish. Old habits are hard to break, so take your time in changing your diet habits so you won't slip back into your old way of eating. However, if this happens, make your health care provider aware as soon as possible, so you can be assisted in getting back on track. Nutritional supplements may be needed to assist you to get back on track by reducing cravings, etc.

FOODS TO EAT AND NOT EAT—
THE PAGE FUNDAMENTAL DIET

Proteins: Eat small amounts of proteins frequently. It is best if you have some protein at each meal. It need not be a large amount at any one time; in fact, it is best if you stick to smaller amounts—2-4 ounces of meat, fish (fresh wild, not farm raised), foul or eggs at a time. Both animal and vegetarian sources of protein are beneficial. Choose a variety of meat products and try to find the healthiest options available (i.e., free range, antibiotic free and/or organic) whenever possible. Eggs, for most people, are an excellent source of protein. Eat the whole egg; the lecithin in the yolk is essential to lowering blood fat and improving liver and brain function.

With any protein, the way in which you prepare it, according to Dr. Melvin Page, is critical. He felt that the closer to raw or rare, the better proteins are for you. That's because any time meats and vegetables are heated over 110° Fahrenheit, crucial enzymes are damaged and lost. Avoid frying. Grilled, boiled, steamed, soft boiled or poached are best. However, with the rise in food-borne sickness, do make sure the tissue does not have excessive red juice from undercooking.

Vegetables: Eat more, more, more! This is the one area where most everyone can improve their diet, and it is an especially important area for you. Always look for a variety, although make the green leafy type your consistent preference. This includes spinach, chard, beet greens, kale, broccoli, mustard greens and so on. Minimize starchy veggies like potatoes and squashes.

As stated above for proteins, the quality of your produce (fresh and organic preferred) and the method of preparation is critical. Raw is preferred with lightly steamed or sautéed as your second choice for all vegetables. Use only butter or olive oil to sauté. When eating salads, try not to eat iceberg lettuce; instead, use lettuce with a rich green color like romaine, sprouts, spinach and raw nuts. Do not make salads your only choice for veggies.

Fruits: Most people wrongly try to drink their fruits. Fruit juice is loaded with the simple sugar fructose, which is shunted into forming triglycerides and, ultimately, stored as fat. Without the fiber in the fruit, juice sends a rapid burst of fructose into the bloodstream. When you do eat fruit: First, only eat one type of fruit at a time on an empty stomach. Second, avoid the sweetest fruits / tropical fruits, except papaya, which is very rich in digestive enzymes (fruits from colder climates are preferred). And third, when possible, eat only the highest quality, fresh and organic fruits. I recommend that my patients eat pears, plums and apples since, as we discussed in the adrenal chapter, they do not negatively impact the adrenal glands and blood sugar.

Carbohydrates: This is a very tricky area. Most people have one classification of carbs when, in reality, there are really three different types: complex, simple and processed. Unfortunately, for most patients suffering with imbalance problems, almost any carbohydrate is a no-no. It is a physiological fact that the more carbohydrates you eat, the more you will want. Craving carbohydrates is a symptom of an imbalance; you can use this craving to monitor your progress. Overall, eat vegetables as your carbohydrate choice and limit grains (even the whole grains can be trouble). When you do eat whole grains, only have them in moderation, and only at dinner. If you start the day with carbohydrates, you are most likely to crave them throughout the day and then you will eat more and it is downhill from there. We've touched upon the dark side to processed carbohydrates in this book—the connection to weight gain, elevated cholesterol and triglycerides, heart disease and cancer. Absolutely stay away from white breads, muffins, cookies, candies, crackers, pastas, white rice and most baked goods.

Wheat and Grains: There has been a tremendous amount of debate regarding grains. Whole unprocessed grains can be rich sources of vitamins and minerals, but *with* soil depletion and the special strains of grain that modern agriculture has developed, it is not clear what nutrients remain. The two predominantly used grains in this country are genetically engineered and have five times the gluten content and only one-third of the protein content of the original wheat from which they were derived. This high gluten content is to blame for many patients' allergic reactions. I have discovered that omega-3 oils tend to be lacking in those who have gluten sensitivity issues.

When scholars have studied disease patterns and the decline of various civilizations, they found that many of the degenerative diseases developed when cultivation of grains became a major part of their diets. Chemicals naturally found in certain grains, lack of the appropriate enzymes and the carbohydrate content of grains make them a source of trouble for many individuals. My advice at this time is to minimize grains such as wheat, rye and barley. Unprocessed, steel-cut, no-gluten oats and brown rice can be considered on occasion to give you more variety. Some of the Danish and German brown breads, like pumpernickel, seem to be nutritious.

Sweeteners: Use only a *small* amount of raw Tupelo honey or stevia as a sweetener. Absolutely NO NutraSweet®, Splenda®, corn syrup or table sugar. Although Dr. Page did not allow raw sugar cane, it does provide the nutrients to aid in its metabolism. If you decide to deviate, be smart and use only small amounts with a meal.

Fats: The bad news is that you probably do not get enough of the right fats in your diet. Please use olive oil (cold-pressed, extra virgin), walnut oil, flaxseed and grapeseed oils. (Do not heat flax oil). These are actually beneficial, as long as they are cold-pressed.

When cooking, use only raw butter and olive oil. They are the only two oils that it is safe to cook with. Avoid all hydrogenated and partially hydrogenated fats! As we have discussed, these are trans fats and **are poisons to your system!** Never eat margarine again! Also avoid peanut butter; it has the potential to increase mold and yeast in your system. Patients who tend to have chronic sinus challenges tend to eat peanut butter often during the week. Eat all the avocados and raw walnuts, almonds and cashews you desire.

If you think eating fat will make you fat, think again. When you eat fat, a chemical signal is sent to your brain to slow down the movement of food out of your stomach. As a result, you feel full. It is not surprising that recent research is showing that those who eat "fat-free" products tend to actually consume more calories than those who eat foods that have not had their fat content reduced (low in fat usually means high in sugar and/or calories). In addition, fats are used not only for energy, but also for building the membrane around every single cell in your body. Fats also play a role in the formation of hormones, which of course make you feel and function well. It is far worse to be hormone-depleted from a low-fat diet than it is to overeat fat. The sickest patients I see are the ones who have been on a fat-free diet for a long period of time. Like carbohydrates, choose your fats wisely—this program is not suggesting fried or processed foods.

Milk Products: Forget *pasteurized* cow milk products (milk, certain cheeses, half and half, ice cream, cottage cheese and yogurt). If you only knew all the potential problems caused by pasteurized milk, you would swear off it forever. Dr. Page found out that milk was actually more detrimental than sugar for many people (man is the only mammal that continues to drink milk after weaning). Avoiding dairy will make it much easier for you to attain your optimal level of health and hormonal balance. *Raw* butter and Kefir (liquid yogurt), however, are excellent sources of essential nutrients and vitamins. Goat and sheep raw cheeses and milk products are great alternatives because their genetic code and fat content are apparently more similar to those of humans than cow milk products are. However, we should still be cautious using these.

There has been a lot of hype about using soy milk and rice milk to replace dairy. While they sound like healthy alternatives, they really are highly processed foods that are primarily simple carbohydrates. You are better off doing without these as well. Of course, Vitamite®, Mocha Mix® and other dairy substitutes are highly processed, nutrient-depleted products that honestly should not be considered a food. Men should not ever use soy; almond milk is turning out to be a great alternative to dairy products.

Liquids: Water is best and then herbal tea. You should drink a minimum of one quart of water a day. Avoid all soda. I would limit coffee. Fruit juices are forbidden because of their high fructose content and dumping of sugar into the bloodstream. An occasional glass of freshly made organic vegetable juice with a meal is probably okay, but water really is best. I would suggest no more than eight ounces of fresh juice at a time, then eat some protein and fat, such as almonds or almond butter, which will shut off the release of insulin and then cortisol.

If you enjoy wine or beer and still insist on drinking them, there are some guidelines. First, drink only with meals; organic wine is now available and a great option. Red wine has less sugar and more of the beneficial polyphenols than white wines. Most of the good foreign beer is actually brewed and contains far more nutrients than the pasteurized chemicals called "beer" made by the large commercial breweries in the United States. Less is better. Drink these occasionally rather than regularly. Because coffee and alcohol force you to lose water (called diuretics), you will have to drink more water to compensate. Personally, I would eliminate alcohol.

The most important life-giving substance in the body is water. The daily routine of the body depends on a turnover of about 40,000 glasses of water per day. In the process, your body loses a minimum of 6 glasses per day, even if you do nothing other than breathe. With movement, exercise and sugar intake (that's right), you can require up to 15 glasses of water per day. Consider this—the concentration of water in your brain has been estimated to be 85 percent; the water content of your tissues, like your liver, kidney, muscle, heart, intestines, and so on, is 75 percent water. The concentration of water outside of the cells is about 94 percent. That means that the water wants to move from the outside of the cell (diluted) into the cell (more concentrated) to balance out things. The urge water has to move is called hydroelectric power. That is the same electrical power generated at hydroelectric dams (like the Hoover Dam). The energy made in your body is in part hydroelectric. There is no one who couldn't use a little boost of energy—so drink more water!

EAT SMALLER AMOUNTS MORE FREQUENTLY

Eating a smaller amount reduces the stress of digestion on your energy supply. Eating small meals conserves energy. Give your energy generator a chance to keep up with digestion by not overwhelming it with a large meal. The average mealtime in the United States is 15 minutes long. In Europe, the average mealtime is one to one and a half hours. It's little wonder Americans suffer such a high rate of digestive disorders! When digestion is impaired, yeast overgrowth, gas, inflammation and food reactions are the results.

Another reason for eating smaller meals is to prevent the ups and downs of your blood sugar level, so you end up craving less sugar. As mentioned earlier, you can overwhelm your digestive capacity. You can also subvert your body's ability to handle sugar in the blood. Since the body will not (or should not) allow the blood sugar level to get too high, insulin and other hormones are secreted to lower the blood sugar. Oftentimes, the insulin response is too strong and, within a short period of time, insulin has driven the blood sugar level down. As a result of low blood sugar, you get a powerful craving for sugar or other carbohydrates. You then usually overeat, and the cycle of ups and downs, yo-yo blood sugar levels result. Depression and the lack of energy are all part of this cycle. Eating a small meal again will virtually stop this cycle.

Eating smaller meals also has advantages for your immune response to ingested food. It turns out that a small amount of food enters the blood without first going through the normal digestive pathway by way of your liver. As a result, this food is seen by the body not as nourishment, but as a threat that will stimulate an immune reaction. Normally, a small immune reaction is not even noticed, but if a large amount of food is eaten (or if a food is eaten over and over again), the immune reaction can cause symptoms. Over time, disease will develop.

By eating smaller amounts, the size of the reaction that occurs is small and inconsequential. A large meal, and thus a large assault of the immune system, could cause many symptoms of an activated immune system, including fatigue, joint aches, flu-like symptoms, headaches and more. This reaction was called the Metabolic Rejectivity Syndrome by the late nutritional pioneer Arthur L. Kaslow, MD. Through thousands of his patients' food diaries, he compiled a list of high-risk foods that is much the same as Dr. Page's.

Important Note: When in doubt, don't eat it. If it isn't on the list, wait and ask your doctor or nutritionist on your next visit. The Page Diet Plan is designed to help you reach optimal health as it has for tens of thousands of Dr. Page's patients. Many are in their later years without signs of degenerative diseases, such as heart disease, arthritis, cancer, osteoporosis, etc. It is not intended to make you suffer or sacrifice. Quite the opposite is true, as you will be delighted with the physical and emotional improvements you experience from the food your body was designed to run on optimally. And what you eat and drink at the occasional party or evening out is not going to be significantly harmful to your nutritional balance in the long run. So go ahead and enjoy—but very moderately.

Lastly, as with all things that are beneficial to your health, it is hard to start, but the longer you use this diet, the greater the benefits you will realize from it. Relax and enjoy the benefits!

Each of your meals must include some protein. the easiest sources are meat, fish, poultry or eggs. (Count 2 eggs as equal to 3 oz.) Vegetarians must combine proteins carefully and consistently using a different calculation. An easy way to calculate the amount of protein you need is to divide your ideal body weight by 15 to get the number of ounces of protein to be consumed per day. This is not a "high protein diet." Like many people, you already eat this much protein during a day, but you eat it mostly in one or two meals instead of spreading it out evenly over three to five meals. If you are more physically active, eat more protein.

90 lb. IBW = 6 oz. per day or 1¾ – 2 oz. of protein per serving.
105 lb. IBW = 7 oz. per day or 1¾ – 2⅓ oz. of protein per serving.
120 lb. IBW = 8 oz. per day or 2 – 2¾ oz. of protein per serving.
135 lb. IBW = 9 oz. per day or 2½ – 3 oz. of protein per serving.
150 lb. IBW = 10 oz. per day or 3 – 3⅓ oz. of protein per serving.
165 lb. IBW = 11 oz. per day or 3⅓ – 3¾ oz. of protein per serving.

I would like to explain how to use the following food guides. The chart's basis is on the glycemic index, which was discussed in Chapter 16. Phase I focuses on items that are lower in the glycemic index. They will affect your blood sugar more slowly, creating a steady flow of blood sugar rather than spikes that create an insulin rush. The vegetables listed are loaded with minerals, especially if you focus on organic-sourced products. These particular foods will assist your body in the utilization of the protein you are consuming.

When two weeks or so have passed, you can then add Phase II, which has veggies that have a higher glycemic index number, meaning they will stimulate a bit more insulin and get the blood glucose into the cells quicker. Personally, I avoid the 12-21 percent carbs group in

Phase II. I would strongly encourage you to only eat the fruits on the list. I have found that people in our culture have major health challenges because they focus too much on sweet fruits.

PHASE I FOOD PLAN
FOR BALANCING BODY CHEMISTRY
PROTEINS: MEAT — FISH — FOWL — EGGS
(SEE PROTEIN CHART FOR INDIVIDUAL PORTION SIZE, PAGE 246)

VEGETABLES: (No Limit on Serving Size)

VEGETABLES 3% OR LESS CARBS	VEGETABLES 6% OR LESS CARBS	VEGETABLES 7 – 9% CARBS	OTHER FOODS IN LIMITED AMOUNTS
ASPARAGUS	BELL PEPPERS	ACORN SQUASH	BUTTER, RAW
BAMBOO SHOOTS	BOK CHOY STEMS	ARTICHOKES	CAVIAR
BEAN SPROUTS	CHIVES	AVOCADO	COTTAGE CHEESE, RAW
BEET GREENS	EGGPLANT	BEETS	DRESSING – OIL / CIDER VINEGAR ONLY
BOK CHOY	GREEN BEANS	BRUSSEL SPROUTS	JERKY
GREENS	GREEN ONIONS	BUTTERNUT SQUASH	KEFIR, RAW (LIQUID YOGURT)
BROCCOLI	OKRA	CARROTS	MILK, RAW
CABBAGES	OLIVES	JICAMA	NUTS, RAW (EXCEPT PEANUTS)
CAULIFLOWER	PICKLES	LEEKS	OILS – VEGETABLE, OLIVE (NO CANOLA)
CELERY	PIMENTO	ONION	PREFERABLY COLD-PRESSED
CHARDS	RHUBARB	PUMPKIN	
CHICORY	SWEET POTATOES	RUTABAGAS	**BEVERAGES**
COLLARD GREENS	TOMATOES	TURNIPS	BEEF TEA
CUCUMBER	WATER CHESTNUTS	WINTER SQUASHES	BOUILLON – BEEF, CHICKEN
ENDIVE	YAMS		HERBAL (DECAFFEINATED) TEAS
ESCAROLE			FILTERED OR SPRING WATER
GARLIC			
KALE			
KOHLRABI			
LETTUCES			
MUSHROOMS			
MUSTARD GREENS			
PARSLEY			
RADISHES			
RAW COB CORN			
SALAD GREENS			
SAUERKRAUT			
SPINACH			
STRING BEANS			
SUMMER SQUASHES			
TURNIP GREENS			
WATERCRESS			
YELLOW SQUASH			
ZUCCHINI SQUASH			

■ FOODS EATEN CLOSEST TO THEIR RAW STATE HAVE THE BEST DIGESTIVE ENZYME ABILITY.
■ TAKE FLUIDS MORE THAN ONE HOUR BEFORE OR MORE THAN TWO HOURS AFTER MEALS.
■ LIMIT FLUID INTAKE WITH MEALS TO NO MORE THAN 4 OZ.
■ NO PROCESSED GRAINS, WHITE FLOUR, SUGAR, SUGAR SUBSTITUTES.

PHASE II FOOD PLAN
FOR BALANCING BODY CHEMISTRY

PROTEINS: MEAT — FISH — FOWL — EGGS
(SEE PROTEIN CHART FOR INDIVIDUAL PORTION SIZE, PAGE 246)

VEGETABLES: (No Limit on Serving Size)

VEGETABLES 3% OR LESS CARBS	VEGETABLES 6% OR LESS CARBS	VEGETABLES 12 – 21% CARBS	OTHER FOODS IN LIMITED AMOUNTS
ASPARAGUS	BELL PEPPERS	ON LIMITED BASIS	BUTTER, RAW
BAMBOO SHOOTS	BOK CHOY STEMS	(ONLY 2-3 X/WEEK)	CAVIAR
BEAN SPROUTS	CHIVES	ARTICHOKES	COTTAGE CHEESE, RAW
BEET GREENS	EGGPLANT	CELERIAC	DRESSING – OIL / CIDER VINEGAR ONLY
BOK CHOY	GREEN BEANS	CHICKPEAS	JERKY
GREENS	GREEN ONIONS	COOKED CORN	KEFIR, RAW (LIQUID YOGURT)
BROCCOLI	OKRA	GRAINS, SPROUTED	MILK, RAW
CABBAGES	OLIVES	HORSERADISH	NUTS, RAW (EXCEPT PEANUTS)
CAULIFLOWER	PICKLES	KIDNEY BEANS	OILS – VEGETABLE, OLIVE (NO CANOLA)
CELERY	PIMENTO	LIMA BEANS	PREFERABLY COLD-PRESSED
CHARDS	RHUBARB	LENTILS	
CHICORY	SWEET POTATOES	PARSNIPS	
COLLARD GREENS	TOMATOES	PEAS	
CUCUMBER	WATER CHESTNUTS	POTATOES	
ENDIVE	YAMS	SEEDS, SPROUTED	
ESCAROLE		SUNFLOWER SEEDS	
GARLIC			
KALE			

VEGETABLES 3% OR LESS CARBS	VEGETABLES 7 – 9% CARBS	FRUITS	BEVERAGES
KOHLRABI			
LETTUCES			
MUSHROOMS	ACORN SQUASH	LIMITED QUANTITY	BEEF TEA
MUSTARD GREENS	ARTICHOKES	ON LIMITED BASIS	BOUILLON – BEEF, CHICKEN
PARSLEY	AVOCADO	(SNACKS ONLY)	HERBAL (DECAFFEINATED) TEAS
RADISHES	BEETS	APPLES	FILTERED OR SPRING WATER
RAW COB CORN	BRUSSEL SPROUTS	BERRIES	RED WINE ONLY (3 GLASSES MAX)
SALAD GREENS	BUTTERNUT SQUASH	GRAPES PAPAYA	
SAUERKRAUT	CARROTS JICAMA	PEARS PRUNES,	DESSERT
SPINACH	LEEKS	FRESH	
STRING BEANS	ONION		PLAIN GELATIN ONLY
SUMMER	PUMPKIN		
SQUASHES	RUTABAGAS		
TURNIP GREENS	TURNIPS		
WATERCRESS	WINTER SQUASHES		
YELLOW SQUASH			
ZUCCHINI SQUASH			

- FOODS EATEN CLOSEST TO THEIR RAW STATE HAVE THE BEST DIGESTIVE ENZYME ABILITY.
- TAKE FLUIDS MORE THAN ONE HOUR BEFORE OR MORE THAN TWO HOURS AFTER MEALS.
- LIMIT FLUID INTAKE WITH MEALS TO NO MORE THAN 4 OZ.
- NO PROCESSED GRAINS, WHITE FLOUR, SUGAR, SUGAR SUBSTITUTES.

THE PAGE FUNDAMENTAL DIET PLAN – ACTION STEPS

I suggest that you read the Page Diet slowly and analyze what you are eating. You will only get the progress you want and expect by making changes and following the guidelines. If sweets are your challenge, focus on eating more complex carbohydrates sourced from veggies. Those items will stabilize sweet cravings. You may need to seek a whole-food source of chromium and Celtic Sea Salt®, which will also help reduce sugar cravings.

Following is an example of what I generally eat during the day:

- ☐ Start the day with warm or hot water with a wedge of lemon; sip the water and eat the lemon pulp, as this promotes digestion and liver health.

- ☐ For breakfast, have half of an apple with almond butter, a scrambled egg with grilled veggies or a piece of grilled chicken or turkey. You can't go wrong with veggies and protein, but I would not eat cereal. If you desire a grain, try quinoa.

- ☐ Create a bag of veggies to eat throughout the day: four or five carrots, small tomatoes, one half of an apple, slices of radishes, cucumber slices and celery. I eat a bag of veggies every day.

- ☐ Take a bag of raw and/or roasted nuts with you every day: almonds, cashews and walnuts. Eat these throughout the day when you are hungry.

- ☐ For lunch, have a mixed green salad with protein, such as chicken, turkey or lamb.

- ☐ Have nuts and veggies for an afternoon snack.

- ☐ For dinner, have veggies and chicken, turkey or lamb.

- ☐ As beverages throughout the day, stick to only herbal teas and water.

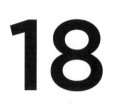

YOUR TRANSITION

Have you ever heard the saying, "Good, better, best. Never let it rest until good becomes better and better becomes best"? This is the best approach to changing the way you and your family eat. Change will come, but it will come little by little. It is a process. The following are excellent transitional charts to assist you in making the transition from good to better to best. This information was taken in part from Junk Food to Real Food: A Blueprint for Healthier Eating by Carol A. Nostrand.

TRANSITION CHART I

FOODS TO AVOID PROTEINS	FOODS TO ENJOY PROTEINS	
ELIMINATE IMMEDIATELY	**ACCEPTABLE FOODS** *EXPERIMENT WITH THESE*	**VITAL FOODS** *PRIMARILY USE THESE*
Meats with additives such as luncheon meat, packed with nitrites (bologna, salami, etc.),	Meat without additives, hormones, antibiotics, etc., raised free-range on organic feed	Sprouts Fresh, raw nuts and seeds: flax, chia, pumpkin, sunflower, sesame, almond, pecan, brazil, walnut, filbert, etc. Nut butters Nut milks Organic eggs
Meat with hormones, etc	Deep ocean or pure-lake fish	
Processed cheese	Nuts and grain as the source to make rice, almond milk, cheese, and yogurt	
Processed eggs		
Processed chicken		
Raised in small coops, injected with antibiotics, etc.	Goat's milk, chevre, feta cheese (Goat's milk is very close to human milk constituents) and is acceptable, but not daily	
Pork		
Pasteurized, homogenized cow's milk	Meat without additives, hormones, antibiotics, etc., raised free-range on organic feed	
Yogurt with sugar, and toxic additives		

TRANSITION CHART II

Foods to Avoid CARBOHYDRATES	Foods to Enjoy CARBOHYDRATES	
Eliminate Immediately	*Acceptable Foods* *Experiment with These*	*Vital Foods* *Primarily Use These*
Sugar: white, brown, turbinado, sucrose, glucose, corn syrup, fructose, etc. Chocolate Processed carbohydrates such as white flour and white flour products White rice Anything packaged or canned with sugar, salt or toxic additives Processed pasta Ice cream with sugar and toxic additives	Raw honey; blackstrap molasses; barley malt pure maple syrup WHOLE GRAIN BREAD Whole grain pasta Grain/Nut ice cream made without toxic additives or sugar	Vegetables: squash, carrots, celery, tomatoes, beets, cabbage, broccoli, cauliflower, leeks, turnips, radishes, lettuce, etc. Fruit: apples, pears, plums, etc. Sea vegetables Whole grains: brown rice millet, rye, barley,etc.

TRANSITION CHART III

FOODS TO AVOID LIPIDS	FOODS TO ENJOY LIPIDS	
ELIMINATE IMMEDIATELY	*ACCEPTABLE FOODS* *EXPERIMENT WITH THESE*	*VITAL FOODS* *PRIMARILY USE THESE*
Oils that are rancid or overheated Rancid animal fats, such as lard, bacon drippings, etc. Anything deep-fat fried Artificially hardened fats, such as margarine and shortenings	High Oleic safflower, sunflower, olive oil Butter	Raw, cold-processed oils: olive, coconut, sesame, flax, almond, walnut, avocado Raw, unsalted butter Avocado Fresh, raw nuts and seeds

TRANSITION CHART IV

FOODS TO AVOID OTHER	FOODS TO ENJOY OTHER	
ELIMINATE IMMEDIATELY	ACCEPTABLE FOODS EXPERIMENT WITH THESE	VITAL FOODS PRIMARILY USE THESE
Coffee, tannic-acid teas; excess alcohol Any commercial condiments with sugar, salt or toxic additives Commercial soft drinks made with toxic additives and sugar	Pure grain coffee substitutes Not more than one glass a day of non-chemicalized wine or beer Aluminum-free baking powder Soft drinks made without chemicals, sugar or toxic additives Potassium balance salt; celtic sea salt Vegetable salt and kelp	Herb teas and seasonings Organic apple cider vinegar Home-made condiments without salt or sugar Fresh juice vegetables and fruits Reverse osmosis purified water Common table salt (sodium chloride)

YOUR TRANSITION – ACTION STEPS

☐ Log your daily food consumption for one week and look at the number of foods in the different categories.

☐ Do not throw away any food items in your pantry. Instead, as you grocery shop, systematically replace the food categories with the quality and type of items you need to change to get healthier. This will make your transition more gradual and therefore long lasting.

☐ Focus on eating whole foods that are not processed.

☐ Step out and try new food items.

☐ Create a list of items you know you want to add, and buy them when they are on sale.

☐ Create a family fun plan and shop with the entire family.

☐ Be creative and experiment with preparing meals at home. You can lower your food budget by nearly 50 percent by "doing it yourself."

NOTES

Chapter 3

1 *Annals of Internal Medicine* 131 (1999): 348–51.

Chapter 4

1 *Obesity Research* 12 (2004): A23.

Chapter 5

1 Center for Science in the Public Interest, "Researchers Failed to Gauge COX-2 Heart-Attack Risks, Despite Early Warnings," *Nutrition Action Healthletter* (February 16, 2005), http://cspinet.org/integrity/press/200502161.html.

Chapter 6

1 "Six Years of Fast-Food Fats Supersizes Monkeys," *New Scientist* 2556 (June 17, 2006): 21.

2 The basis for the information in this chapter has been taken from *The 7 Principles of Fat Burning*, by Eric E. Berg, DC.

Chapter 8

1 Lindsey Galloway and Elizabeth Marglin, "Beauty with a Conscience," *Natural Solutions* (October 1, 2008), http://www.naturalsolutionsmag.com/articles-display/15452/Beauty-With-a-Conscience.

2 Wendy Koch and Elizabeth Weise, "Limits on toxic perchlorate to be set for tap water," *USA Today* (February 3, 2011), http://www.usatoday.com/tech/science/2011-02-03-perchlorate03_ST_N.htm.

3 Center for Science in the Public Interest, *Nutrition Action Healthletter* (April 2008).

Chapter 9

1 Hari Sharma, James Meade, and Rama Misha, *The Answer to Cancer* (New York: Select Books, 2002).

2 Ibid.

3 Women's Health Initiative, U.S. Government (2003).

4 Liz Szabo, "Breast Cancer: Fewer Cases as Older Women Turn from Hormone Therapy," *USA Today* (December 24, 2007), http://www.usatoday.com/news/health/2007-12-23-year-end-breast-cancer_n.htm.

Chapter 10

1 Parker-Pope, "Health Matters: Is Your Wife Pushing You To See a Doctor? Read This -- And Go." *Wall Street Journal* (May 12, 2007).

2 Erectile dysfunction has nothing to do with the potency or presence of sperm. A man may be completely fertile though unable to arrive at an erection or maintain an adequate erection for penetration.

3 Alcohol initially provokes desire but then inhibits the ability to physically follow through.

4 A list of environmental toxins can be obtained from the American Cancer Society's web page, http://www.cancer.org/.

5 Mary Brophy Marcus, "New Study Links Pain Relievers to Erectile Dysfunction." *USA Today* (March 2, 2011).

6 Daniel Mowery, *The Scientific Validation of Herbal Medicine* (Lincolnwood, IL: Keats Publishing, 1986).

7 Elevated cholesterol levels are not the primary cause of heart attacks; many people who suffer a heart attack have normal cholesterol levels. Inflammation of the vessel wall is the primary cause of heart distress.

8 I discuss the role of cholesterol in great detail in *Dr. Bob's Trans Fat Survival Guide.*

9 Read more about the zinc taste test at **www.druglessdoctor.com** under Client Services/Testing Services.

Chapter 12

1 Women who have had a total hysterectomy or are in menopause may still have a hormonal cycle even if they have stopped menstruating.

Chapter 13

1 It's important to understand that avoiding red meat, cheese and saturated fat may help reduce cholesterol, but a sugary diet and the inability to handle stress will continue to keep cholesterol levels elevated.

2 As noted previously, the use of medication to treat high blood pressure can result in erectile dysfunction.

Chapter 17

1 A major portion of the material for this chapter has been provided to the author by the International Foundation for Nutrition and Health (IFNH) and is used with permission. Contact IFNH at the following:

International Foundation for Nutrition and Health
3963 Mission Blvd, San Diego, CA 92109
www.IFNH.org
1.858.288.2533

PRODUCT INQUIRY

There are many companies that create excellent products. I have personally used and have recommended the items mentioned in this book with consistent success. You may in fact have a source of items that have produced the health restoration results you have used to help yourself and / or others if you are a health care provider. I would encourage you to use what you have found successful, but, if you are like so many who come into my office with boxes and bags of partially used bottles and have experienced minimal or no improvement, maybe it is time to seek other options.

If this is your first time thinking about incorporating a drugless natural strategy to achieve optimal health, before you spend your time and money it would be in your best interests to find a knowledgeable, experienced drugless health care provider to assist you in navigating all the possibilities. If you have been pursuing natural care for some time and have either reached a plateau or are not getting the response you desire, do not give up. You would be wise to pursue another provider or contact me to help you. I intentionally did not list a specific protocol for the conditions and body signals I discussed because you and your physiology are as unique as your fingerprint, requiring items precisely for your findings.

You can locate many items such as the castor oil pack and pH paper at a local health or natural food store. I have recommended products from the companies listed below with great success. The source and quality of the items you incorporate do make quite a difference.

If you are unable to locate the products, you can call 1.888.922.5672 or go online at **www.druglessdoctor.com**.

I recommend the following nutritional manufacturers:

- Omega Nutrition
- The Grain and Salt Company (Selina Naturally)

CONSULTATIONS AND SERVICES

I frequently am asked to answer questions in regards to conditions individuals are not receiving answers for. Before contacting me, first exhaust your local health care provider community. If you are not able to receive answers, then have a phone consultation with me or one of my associates. We also have patients travel to our clinic. You can visit my website at **www.druglessdoctor.com** for details. Procedures including hair analysis, saliva testing and other screens can be completed long distance. You would follow the same procedure as you would for a consultation, since these services would need to be sent to the appropriate lab.

SEMINARS-WORKSHOPS-WELLNESS EVENTS
BUSINESSES-CHURCHES-ORGANIZATIONS

I am available on a limited basis to travel to your location. There is time schedule and attendance minimums required. I generally need to schedule six months to one year out, so if you are thinking about having a special event please contact me early, 1-888-922-5672 or email **drbob@druglessdoctor.com.**

INDEX

D

E

F

J

Jacobsen, Steve, 147
Journal of Urology, The, 146
juices, 104
Junk Food to Real Food: A Blueprint for Healthier Eating, 251

K

Kaslow, Dr. Arthur, 245
Kefir, 242
kelp tablet supplements, 27
kidney distress
    symptoms, 114
kidney stones, 196

L

label-reading, 118
laxatives, 213
LDL low-density lipoprotein, 20, 27, 39, 40, 69, 100, 213
leg cramps, 212
LePore, NP, Donald, 26
libido, 165, 176, 183, 185, 204, 208
    decreased, 204
licorice root, 44
lifestyle modifications, 153
linoleic acid, 51, 57, 100
lipids, 39
lipoproteins, 39
liver disease, 33, 34, 151
liver distress, 114
liver function, 78, 113–125
    decreased, 205
    foods to help, 115, 116
    signs of overworking, 116, 117
    stress, 207
liver or big belly body type, 81
liver/gallbladder detoxification system, 80
lobelia, 46
loss in bone mass, 191
    see also osteoporosis
low blood pressure, 43, 44, 201
low blood sugar, 196, 245
low magnesium, 187
low thyroid body signals, 212
low thyroid function, 211
lunch suggestions, 105, 106
lymph nodes, 135
lymphatic system, 134

M

maca root, 153, 176, 201, 209
magnesium, 187
male hormones, 10–12
maltodextrin, 225
maltose, 227, 228
mannitol, 226
maple sugar, 233
maple syrup, 228, 229, 233
margarine, 20, 54, 70, 98, 242
Marglin, Elizabeth, 118
marine-sourced oil, 30, 99
masturbation, 175
melatonin, 4
menopause, 203
menstruation, 176
metabolic rejection syndrome, 245
metabolism, 211, 213
mid-body fat gain, 204
mineralocorticoids, 186, 187
Mocha Mix, 243
monounsaturated fat, 97
mood swings, 176, 203
multi-grain pancakes, 103
mung beans, 148
muscle cramping, 187
muscle pain syndrome, 34
muscle strength, 1
muscle weakness, 204
mutagens, 139

N

Natural Solutions, 118
natural sweeteners
    see sweeteners
nerve compression, 154
nerve damage from surgery, 144
nervous tension, 189
New England Journal of Medicine, 134
niacinamide, 45
Nick, Dr. Gina, 33
nicotine,
    see tobacco use
Nicotine Relief, 45
nocturnal erections, 153
non-steroidal anti-inflammatory drugs (NSAIDs), 147
norepinephrine, 186
normal weight maintenance, 77–95
normalizing hormonal system, 82–85
Nostrand, Carol A., 251

BOOKS BY DR. BOB

DR. BOB'S DRUGLESS GUIDE TO DETOXIFICATION

This may be the most toxic time in history. Daily headlines report the negative conditions of our water, food, and air. The "green movement" is popularly creating a mindset to secure a safer, cleaner environment, but little is said about the circumstances our bodies have to contend with. This book is a logical plan that establishes true wellness in your body from the inside out. Dr. Bob shares clinically proven, time-tested protocols that can be followed in the comfort of your own home—no need to travel to expensive clinics or follow strict and stressful diet plans.

You will learn what to purchase at your own grocery store to maintain a healthy body, be empowered to make wise choices and not be dependent on medications, avert possible surgical intervention to remove an exhausted dysfunctional organ, and learn what to eat and what to avoid to create an optimally functioning cellular environment!

DR. BOB'S DRUGLESS GUIDE TO BALANCING FEMALE HORMONES

The time tested information is this book is designed to create a state of optimal health in the female hormonal system. Dr. Bob's insight into cell function will empower the reader to make wise choices designed to nourish and detoxify the body with items that can be easily incorporated in a day-to-day routine. You will learn that a clear and clean lymphatic system is important and that a functioning liver is vital for balance. The role of nutrients like iodine and proper oil help create the foundation needed to progress into hormonal maturity without annoying body signals. You will be exposed to the procedures that Dr. Bob has used to transition his patients into feeling great without medication.

DR. BOB'S GUIDE TO STOP ADHD IN 18 DAYS

A Drugless Family Guide to Optimal Health

Anyone can successfully overcome ADHD and Hyperactivity without drugs. This book details how to get your children and family off medications and detrimental junk foods filled with trans fatty acids, dairy products, sugar and preservatives, so that they can have optimal, natural health. This is a simple, effective step-by-step plan that includes adding FLAX OIL and modifying your diet and vitamin/mineral intake. The protocol will improve your nervous system function, and help you overcome behavioral and learning problems. It will improve insomnia, mood swings and irritability. The result will be your body healing itself naturally. Participants in the pilot program saw improvement in only 18 days. NATURALLY!

DR. BOB'S TRANS FAT SURVIVAL GUIDE

Why No Fat, Low Fat, Trans Fat is KILLING YOU!

This book explains the dangers of trans fat, commonly called hydrogenated and partially hydrogenated fat, as well as how to recognize it in everyday foods by properly reading nutritional labels. Along with trans fat, you will learn the different types of fats, which ones are beneficial, and which ones should be used for cooking, baking or eating. Not to leave the reader hanging with questions on how to eliminate dangerous fats and take on a healthier approach to life, there are several sections dealing with how to make those changes, transitioning healthier foods into their eating plan. This book will encourage and empower you to make better choices and learn to live an optimal and healthy life.

DR. BOB'S GUIDE TO OPTIMAL HEALTH

A God-Inspired, Biblically-Based
12 Month Devotional to Natural Health Restoration

The Guide to Optimal Health is a Spirit of the Lord inspired collection of natural health tips. There are 365 daily tips designed to slowly transform your life to the finest health. Experience suggests that it may take up to 21 days to create a new habit. The first of 18 different patterns discussed is water. There are 21 daily natural health tips and associated Bible verses focusing on water. There is a daily **Natural Prescription for Health.** At the end of the guide are several reference tables, including a Food Combining Chart, Glycemic Index, a Good and Not So Good Sweeteners Chart, a pH Chart, and a Transition Food Guide. The information you will learn will empower you to make choices that will have an eternal impact on you, your family and friends.

DR. BOB & DEBBIE'S GUIDE TO SEX AND ROMANCE

Dr. Bob and Debbie's Guide to Sex and Romance is a collection of personal and clinically based evidence including protocols applied and successfully used from Dr. Bob's health care practice. Dr. Bob and Debbie also share from their commonsense experience from 40 years of their personal relationship and over 30 years of marriage. You will gain from the insight they have gleaned from their involvement and observations discovered while being in Natural Health since 1978. The DeMarias have watched the decline of the overall personal health of the new patients presented to the clinic and discuss the restoration of those individuals' overall health. Dr. Bob linked the associated deterioration of sexual desire and whole body dysfunction with patients having chronic health challenges.

Special Appearances
Radio, TV &
Corporate Events

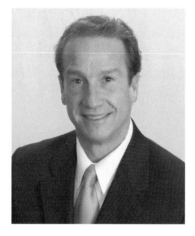

Dr. DeMaria is available on a limited basis to speak at your next Corporate Event or Convention. His energetic speaking style will inspire, educate and motivate your employees or downline to greater levels of health, wealth and personal confidence. Dr. Bob's enthusiasm for life is **contagious!**

To schedule or inquire please call:

1.888.922.5672

or email: drbob@druglessdoctor.com